THE TASK-CENTRED BOOK

Task-centred social work is one of the best known and most strongly supported approaches to social work practice. The model fits well with the long-standing emphasis in social work on empowerment, as well as with more recent pressure for evidence-based practice.

This text is a radical departure from traditional literature on social work methods. The main reference point is the voice of practitioners, service users and carers, as researched and developed by the authors over twenty years. Case studies are used throughout the book to build on the experiences of practitioners and the people with whom they have worked and to demonstrate practical skills for:

- studying and analysing
- teaching and learning
- practising task-centred social work
- review and continuing development.

The Task-Centred Book is a core text for both undergraduate social work courses and continuing professional development training, as well as being a practical book for the active professional which will support the development and implementation of task-centred practice.

Peter Marsh is Professor of Child and Family Welfare, University of Sheffield.

Mark Doel is Research Professor of Social Work, Sheffield Hallam University.

the social work skills series

published in association with *Community Care*

series editor: Terry Philpot

the social work skills series

- builds practice skills step by step
- places practice in its policy context
- relates practice to relevant research
- provides a secure base for professional development

This new, skills-based series has been developed by Routledge and *Community Care* working together in partnership to meet the changing needs of today's students and practitioners in the broad field of social care. Written by experienced practitioners and teachers with a commitment to passing on their knowledge to the next generation, each text in the series features: *learning objectives; case examples; activities to test knowledge and understanding; summaries of key learning points; key references; suggestions for further reading.*

Also available in the series:

Commissioning and Purchasing
Terry Bamford
Executive Director of Housing and Social Services in Kensington and Chelsea. Former Chair of the British Association of Social Workers.

Managing Aggression
Ray Braithwaite
Consultant and trainer in managing aggression at work. Lead trainer and speaker in the national 'No Fear' campaign.

Tackling Social Exclusion
John Pierson
Institute of Social Work and Applied Social Studies, Staffordshire University.

Safeguarding Children and Young People
Corinne May-Chahal and Stella Coleman
Professor of Applied Social Science at Lancaster University and Senior Lecturer in Social Work at the University of Central Lancashire.

THE TASK-CENTRED BOOK

Peter Marsh and Mark Doel

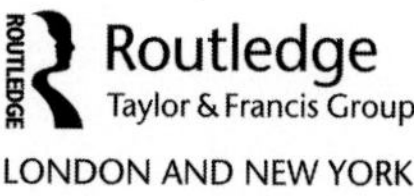

LONDON AND NEW YORK

communitycare

First published 2005 by Routledge
2 Park Square, Milton Park, Abingdon, Oxfordshire, OX14 4RN

Simultaneously published in the USA and Canada
by Routledge
270 Madison Avenue, New York, NY 10016

Routledge is an imprint of the Taylor & Francis Group

Typeset in Sabon and Futura
by J&L Composition, Filey, North Yorkshire
Printed and bound in Great Britain by
TJ International Ltd, Padstow, Cornwall

British Library Cataloguing in Publication Data
A catalogue record for this book is available from the British Library

Library of Congress Cataloging in Publication Data
A catalog record for this book has been requested

ISBN 0-415-33455-1 (hbk)
ISBN 0-415-33456-x (pbk)

To Annie and Jan.

Professor William J. Reid 1928–2003

For over 40 years Bill Reid was the leading light for practice-based research and for the principles which underpin this book. He was an outstanding social scientist and a warm and generous colleague. We owe much to Bill's leadership and wisdom.

CONTENTS

ACTIVITIES

BOXES

ACKNOWLEDGEMENTS

We would like to thank the task-centred practitioners, and the service users and carers they worked with, all of whom have been so central to the development of this book. In particular, our thanks go to Nicola Boyer, Dilani Dresser, Sam Fuller, Dorothy Hand, Carol Harrison, Lisa Hewitt-Craft, Lynne Lawrence, Sarah Lewis, Michelle Lowrie, Kate Race, Catherine Stephenson and Claire Teague.

Our thanks to Steven Appleby (*Guardian* cartoonist) for his permission to use the 'Psychic Cab' cartoon in Chapter 6.

INTRODUCTION

> The family was asked what they thought of this way of working. Diana said she had not had any involvement with social services before, and didn't really know what to expect. She said she didn't expect to be involved in the work, rather that we were going to tell her what was wrong. Diana said that when she contacted social services the only thing she had thought of was Mat's behaviour towards her and his stepfather and she wanted this to stop. Working in this way had given her an opportunity to understand *why* Mat behaved in this way.
>
> (Portfolio D 2002: 5.2)

WHY *THE TASK-CENTRED BOOK*?

There are a number of reasons why we have written this book. The first is that task-centred work fits so many of the developments in social work in recent times, in particular partnership work with service users and evidence-based practice. It feels that task-centred work has come of age.

The second is the growing evidence of the need for more focus on the development of professional practice in social work. There have been important developments in the UK, such as a new council which will register social workers and uphold standards, and a new professional award which means the profession will become solely graduate. However, alongside these developments are the concerns expressed by many social workers that direct work with service users and carers (professional intervention) is becoming relatively marginal to what social workers do, and that the skills of social work are being reduced to an application of a set of administrative procedures, drawn primarily from a substantial agency guidance manual.

The third reason for the book is our joint experience of teaching and developing task-centred work over more than two decades, and the clear indications that knowing about the model is not enough. Knowledge about task-centred work does not easily move into practice activities. It is clear that implementing and supporting task-centred practice is a complex activity, and an essential one, if the learning is to be transferred to regular and sustained practice. We want to plough back the experience of working with social workers to develop professional practice.

SUPPORTING THE DEVELOPMENT OF PRACTICE

This is a book designed to have a real impact on practice. It is based on research carried out by us, and integrated into our training and development work since the early 1980s. A major theme of the book is the significance of supporting practice development. This is a process of innovation which, sadly, often falters beyond the one-off project and fails to make it into mainstream work (Smale 1996).

In this book, we aim to support practice development in general, and task-centred practice in particular, by drawing on the experience of our research and development work with practitioners, managers and their wider agencies over a number of years. Very many of these practitioners (and, indeed, some of their managers) compiled portfolios of their task-centred experiences, providing careful evidence of their learning and practice. We focus on the work of twelve of these practitioners. Their work, alongside that of the service users and carers they were involved with, is central to this book. We hope that the illustrations drawn from their experiences of learning, implementing and developing professional practice will prove an interesting and useful guide for the reader, and a positive aid to developing practice.

The example work has been chosen to span key areas of social work, and also to examine a variety of learning experiences. It provides help with the details of what is to be done, shows particular difficulties and opportunities, and highlights areas for learning, teaching and support. The significance of the context of social work practice is also highlighted through these examples. All names and circumstances have been altered to preserve confidentiality.

Our work in developing and evaluating courses in task-centred practice, and the work of the practitioners, service users and carers themselves, form the backbone of the book. It is a significant development from our previous book on task-centred practice (Doel and Marsh 1992), which will continue to provide an introduction to the task-centred model itself. *The Task-Centred Book* is designed, we hope, to have the greatest likelihood of improving practice by building on the experiences of practitioners and the people with whom they have worked. As such, it is an example of research in practice.

The book is a radical departure from the literature on social work methods. Though we make use of the traditional literature, the book's main reference point is the voice of practitioners, service users and carers, as evidenced through portfolios written and compiled alongside the task-centred work. Certainly, the opportunity to use the testimony from well-constructed portfolios (for not all portfolio formats are reliable) means that practitioners, service users and carers are central to the development of professional practice (Doel *et al.* 2002). We hope this approach will become mainstream to the development of social work practice over the coming years.

STRUCTURE OF THE BOOK

The book develops in a broadly chronological order, providing background to the model, and then increasing detail of it, using different chapters to explore different facets, such as the teaching and learning of the model. As you will appreciate, advice about how to use the book is difficult, since individual readers' circumstances vary so much. However, the book offers a wide variety of ways of learning about task-centred practice and of developing strategies to implement it. We have written the book with a broad constituency of readers in mind, and this is reflected in the activities and boxes. Most chapters can be read on their own, with each providing a different perspective on task-centred practice; some naturally group together (such as Chapters 6 and 7 on do and review). You may want to move from Chapter 3 to Chapters 6 and 7, and read Chapters 4 and 5 on teaching and learning separately. Of course, we hope you will feel encouraged to read the whole book and not just an odd chapter!

Regarding terminology, we have aimed to be gender neutral, preferring the use of 'they' where appropriate. We use the term 'learner' to denote anybody who is learning about task-centred practice; this is a more inclusive term than 'students' (which, in the UK, usually means people who are not yet qualified) and 'candidates' (often used for people who are studying for post-qualification and post-registration awards). 'Learner' also includes people who are not enrolled in any formal programme of study and, of course, it can encompass people who learn about task-centred practice as service users or carers. We use the word 'people' to describe people, but sometimes it is necessary to differentiate people's roles as practitioners, service users or carers.

ACTIVITIES AND BOXES

In common with other books in this series we have used boxes to indicate key points in discrete sections, and we sometimes make reference to boxes that are not in the current chapter (the numbering provides the chapter location and then the box order). Activities provide an additional route of learning for six different groups of people. We have included activities for each of these groups of people in each of the chapters to emphasise the significance of all of these groups in developing good practices. However, most activities have some relevance and interest beyond the particular group mentioned in the activity heading, and we would encourage you to read all the activities and cross boundaries by participating in some from other groups. The six groups are as follows:

- *Service users and carers* who want to help develop the service. We would like to encourage those in direct contact with service users and carers to make use of the book where appropriate, especially in using some of the activities.
- *Learners* who are relatively new to social work practice in general or to task-centred work in particular.
- *Practitioners* who are developing their task-centred work based on existing practice experience. In general this will be social work and social care staff, though the task-centred model can be used by different professions and has the potential to create more co-working between professions.
- *Supervisors* who support staff doing this work.
- *Trainers* who lead training programmes on task-centred practice.
- *Managers* who aim to provide a good learning environment for task-centred practice and ways of embedding it in agency practice.

There are suggested answers for some of the activities in the Appendix.

AN INTRODUCTION TO THE PORTFOLIOS

The level of detail differs in respect of each portfolio presented in this book. Some are prominent and are introduced with a relatively detailed summary (e.g. Box 3.1), most reappear in a number of chapters, and one or two have only a passing reference. Just as it is not necessary to know the plot of a film in order to appreciate a particular cinematographic technique, there are times in the book when detailed background information about a particular situation would obscure the central point in question and clutter the page. However, there will be occasions when readers want to locate the players in a particular situation, so here is the briefest of précis of the twelve situations:

Portfolio A (2000)

Practitioner: Victoria, pre-qualified, working at a Pre-5 Family Centre.
Service user: Sharon, 30s, problems with anger towards child, Tom, 4, and high expectations.

Portfolio B (2002)

Practitioner: Erica, qualified, working in a Community Mental Health team.
Service user: Kelly, 20s, epilepsy, agoraphobia, access to general practitioner (GP); carer Tina (see Box 3.1).

Portfolio C (1995)

Practitioner: Tamsin, qualified, working in a Specialist Child Care Service.
Service user: Mandy, 14, and family – rehabilitation home.

Portfolio D (2002)

Practitioner: Sue, qualified, working in a Children and Families team.
Service user: Diana, 30s, and Mat, 11, and stepbrother Daniel, 12 – physical attacks by Mat on mother.

Portfolio E (2000)

Practitioner: Kathy, pre-qualified, working in Adult Services (Learning Disabilities).
Service user: Dave, 20s, mild learning difficulties wishing to move into independence. Staying temporarily with his sister, Sheila, a single parent with two boys (see Box 2.3).

Portfolio F (2003)

Practitioner: Barbara, qualified, working in a Youth Offending team.
Service user: Wayne, 17, mixed race, a youth offender, and a heroin user; mother, Sue.

Portfolio G (2000)

Practitioner: Andrea, qualified, working in a Children and Families team.
Service user: Evelyn, 30s, children's welfare, school attendance, budgeting problems; eldest son: Carl, 17.

Portfolio H (1996)

Practitioner: Friyana, qualified, working in a Specialist Child Care team.
Service user: Louise, 20s, wants to stop Steven's (her 2-year-old son) tantrums (see Box 2.2).
Service user: Hill/Sarita family (Mr Hill and Mrs Sarita) – marital problems and behaviour of son, Yusef, 9.

Portfolio I (2003)

Practitioner: Laura, pre-qualified, working in Supported Living Services.
Service user: Roger, 30, learning difficulties, autism, wheelchair, choosing drinks.

Portfolio J (2002)

Practitioner: Margaret, qualified, Adults Community team.
Service user: Paula, 29, dependent on mother with terminal illness; bereavement work (Box 3.2).

Portfolio K (2002)

Practitioner: Gwen, pre-qualified, Mental Health Support team.
Service user: John, 54, schizophrenic, poor confidence, wants to go to café on own (Box 3.3).

Portfolio L (2000)

Practitioner: Jane, qualified, Community Mental Health team.
Service user: Dan, mid-20s, drug-induced psychosis, lack of motivation – wants to get out more.

Task-centred work can have a dramatic impact on people's lives. We believe it has a central role in developing professional practice; indeed, many practitioners have described their learning and practice of task-centred work as a reintroduction to what they understood professional social work to be. While playing its part to develop task-centred work, we hope that this book can also support continuing practice development for social work as a whole.

CHAPTER 1

DEVELOPMENT

OBJECTIVES

By the end of this chapter you should:

- Recognise the complex translation of ideas into action in social work practice
- Be able to outline underpinning elements of task-centred practice
- Know about the early development and general outline of task-centred practice
- Understand why task-centred practice is an 'innovation' in practice
- See the challenges and opportunities for the development of task-centred work.

DEVELOPMENT: THE ORIGINS AND BACKGROUND OF TASK-CENTRED PRACTICE

Developing social work practice is a complex and challenging activity. That will be a consistent theme of this book, and this first chapter not only lays much of the groundwork as to why it is complex and challenging, but also describes some key elements that need to be present for the sound development of practice. The importance of service users' and carers' views, the role of science and evidence, and the need to take full account of the diversity of people's lives are all covered here. The origins and basic outline of task-centred practice are presented, together with the ways that this model may be developed, with the challenges and opportunities that are offered to such a development.

WHY STUDY PRACTICE?

Under the general heading 'social work is work with people: it's that simple and that complicated', the UK government explains what social work is, for those thinking of it as a career, as follows:

> Social work is all about people. Social workers form relationships with people. As adviser, advocate, counsellor or listener, a social worker helps people to live more successfully within their local communities by helping them find solutions to their problems. Social work also involves engaging with not only clients themselves but their families and friends as well, as well as working closely with other organisations including the police, NHS, schools and probation service.
>
> (Department of Health 2004)

This range of activities clearly needs some underpinning knowledge, for example the law, policies and regulations, psychology and sociology. But the 'application' of these areas of knowledge, and the 'practical' activity of working with the people involved, and planning and helping with their care and protection, may be thought of, by many, as strongly related to common sense. No doubt in discussions and in arguments, within a family or between friends in a pub, there are views being put forward about the right way to advise people or to 'live more successfully'. Sometimes these discussions might acknowledge the need for some particular information, for example about the law, but they are not likely to stress the need for a study of 'application' or 'practice' for these sorts of activities. The suggestion that learning easily converts into doing may be right in some areas, but definitely not in social work. The conversion process is complex. It's about the law, it's about the people, and it's about the 'stuck' situations that are often brought to social workers.

First, the legal issues are far from straightforward in 'application'. There are issues of power and control, for example, where social workers have to present to service users the legal case for requiring them to do or not do certain things. How do you put this in the way that is likely to be most effective? How can you do it and still allow people choice in areas that are not part of the requirements? How can you do it and still work with people to encourage them to do other things, for example to write to their child in care even if they cannot see their child? These may appear to have common-sense answers, but there are as many common-sense answers as there are people discussing them.

Second, social workers need to see the service user's point of view, and they often need to see many service users' points of view. These views are central: they should drive the actions that are not legally required. For many decades social work has been developing a 'partnership' approach to practice which bases work, as far as possible, on views, wishes and experiences of service users (Marsh and Fisher 1992), and this is now clearly outlined in the statement of ethics or professional code for registered social workers in the UK (General Social Care Council 2002: see Box 2.1). However, working to this principle is not easy. Individual views about care and protection are often strongly held. Within families or groups it is all too common for blame to be allocated and entrenched patterns of misunderstanding to set in. In short there is very likely to be some element of conflict in these views. This conflict will be expressed in the context of the individual's language, religion, 'race' and culture (as the law concerning children in England and Wales puts it (Children Act 1989 s.24). Conflict and multifaceted personal culture make the understanding of views notably complex.

Third, the situations that social workers often work in are usually complex. The situations have usually reached some sort of crisis, or some form of impasse. People are 'stuck', without knowledge of the right actions to take, or without the ability or willingness to act on the knowledge they do have. People do not generally come to social workers with simple problems; they solve those elsewhere. So the issues already mentioned of power and understanding are likely to be taking place in situations that are far from ordinary. Practice in social work is rarely located in ordinary circumstances; these circumstances are nearly always unusual and difficult, probably best described as extra-ordinary. Applying knowledge and listening to service users is substantially more challenging in such circumstances.

Applying the knowledge of child or adult psychology, or the law, or a policy, is not easy. 'Practice' is an important area of study in social work. A social worker is not just a 'lawyer-lite' or a 'psychologist-lite' professional. Social workers need professional practice knowledge and skills of their own, not least to apply the underpinning subject knowledge, some of which will be shared with other professions.

The history of social work has reflected this need, and numerous approaches to practice have been put forward. This book is concerned with one of those approaches: task-centred practice. It will be our argument in these pages that this approach has many reasons to commend it, not least that it directly addresses the three issues outlined above: it is directly concerned with power and compulsion, the need for understanding others, and the need to reduce the complexity of social problems to manageable proportions.

THE BUILDING BLOCKS OF TASK-CENTRED PRACTICE

How then has task-centred practice been built? It has rested on three main pillars: research, service user views and wishes, and practitioner experience.

Practice-based research into effective ways of carrying out the activities needed in social work (with all of the complexities outlined above) has underpinned its development. Studies have researched analysis, planning, doing, and reviewing, and built one on another into a substantial body of work.

The second pillar is the accumulated experience of practitioners, sometimes expressed through research, but often based on practice wisdom because of the possibilities that task-centred work offers for a continuing development of practice *through practice*, a point we will return to later.

The third pillar is that provided by the views and wishes of service users and carers, sometimes expressed via organised processes, such as advocacy groups, sometimes again expressed within research, but more often directly embodied in the practice itself. The view of the service user and carer is at the centre of task-centred practice.

Knowledge-based practice

This tripartite formulation of knowledge has been well expressed by Janet Lewis (2001), who was for many years the research director of the Joseph Rowntree Trust research foundation, which sought to combine research, service user and carer views, and practitioner experience in generating applied knowledge for practice. She entered the complex debates about evidence-based practice (Trinder 2000), where this tripartite base has been expressed in a number of different ways, and suggested a pair of memorable equations. Her formulation was that research could be used as evidence once there had been satisfactory interpretation of the findings. This process of translation needed to be undertaken to convert the raw outcomes of a study into recommendations for action, and it formed the first equation. This evidence then joined the experience of practitioners and the views and wishes of service users and carers in forming the knowledge for practice, and the second equation. These two equations are in Box 1.1, and we will return to the second one in particular a number of times throughout the book.

BOX 1.1: KNOWLEDGE FOR PRACTICE

Evidence = Research 'findings' + interpretation of the findings

Knowledge = Evidence + practice wisdom + service user and carer experience and wishes

Lewis's neat formulation is a good basis for a profession based on putting the views and wishes of service users and carers at its centre, while coupling this with research and with practice experience. It suggests that ideally practitioners could outline the contribution of each of the three elements within the particular knowledge they were using. An entertaining article has noted that not adhering to this ideal may result in some unfortunate alternative models of practice that have remarkably little content . . . see Box 1.2 as a cautionary tale!

BOX 1.2: ALTERNATIVES TO EVIDENCE-BASED PRACTICE?

Noting that there are many circumstances when there is little evidence to guide medical practice, a light-hearted article in the *British Medical Journal* proposed a series of other models which could sometimes be seen in action.

These included

- eminence-based practice – where status counts
- vehemence-based practice – where stridency counts
- eloquence-based practice – where smoothness of tongue counts.

And, suggested as being available to surgeons only, there was also

- confidence-based practice – based purely on bravado.

(Isaacs and Fitzgerald 1999)

While we argue that task-centred practice is especially well placed to put together these three elements of knowledge in the practice context of social work outlined above, nonetheless we appreciate the problems faced in generating such knowledge.

Research into practice has been far too limited in social work. There needs to be a focus directly on the practice activities of social workers, and how they can best respond to the kind of difficulties outlined above. Task-centred literature provides an impressive body of work on this area, but given the centrality of the issue there is remarkably little else (Smale 1983). In part this is due to an under-investment, in the UK at least, in social work and social care research (Fisher and Marsh 2003). Within this under-investment the lack of practice research is also due to the lack of connection between practitioners and researchers (McCartt Hess and Mullen 1995). The limited amount of social care research has generally concentrated on policy, rather than on practice.

Equally the basis in service user and carer wishes and experiences has been, in part, a rocky road. Social work can be proud that there are numerous examples of the voices of service users and carers within research studies, but other aspects of involvement have been a long and hard struggle (Barnes and Bowl 2001). While task-centred work has these views and wishes at its heart there are often likely to be struggles in getting these voices centre stage in all aspects of service.

The voice of practice, directly from practitioners, has also not been heard as much as it might. Practice-based discussions are not that common in social work, despite the evidence of developmental models such as communities of practice which we cover in Chapter 8. Practitioners have not found it easy to talk about practice, and with the *Blackwell Encyclopaedia of Social Work* (Davies 2000) listing 106 'methods' (including 'nothing works') and 42 'theories', it is not surprising that this has proved difficult.

As we argued in the early 1990s, social workers need a language of practice so that they can

> begin to compare notes about what works, when and with whom. They can begin to research their own practice and to involve the users of the social services in this process. Together they can speak with authority about the value of social work.
>
> (Doel and Marsh 1992: x)

It is the strong combination of the voices of service users and carers, practitioners and researchers that makes task-centred work so powerful.

Cultural competence

We noted earlier the complexity of understanding people's views and wishes when they are mediated through the complexities of language, religion, 'race' and culture. Social work has, quite rightly, often paid special attention to these areas, although it has, in common with all other services, also been appallingly neglectful of them at times. It is absolutely right to be concerned with the ways that language, religion, 'race' and culture are key elements in people's lives, and shape and affect their choices, options and desires; and, of course, age, class, sexuality and ability are all part of this equation. To respond appropriately we need to be respectful of others, to challenge discrimination, and to allow ourselves constantly to learn from the aspects of identity that we are dealing with that are different from our own.

> It is often the way we look at other people that imprisons them within their own narrowest allegiances. And it is also the way we look at them that may set them free.
>
> (Maalouf 2000: 19)

An open view, allowing for learning and for creativity, is well reflected in all the aspects of task-centred practice. It is fully appropriate to the multicultural nature of modern Britain (Alibhai-Brown 2001), and it is coming to be an important part of all social work (O'Hagan 2001).

To enact this open and respectful stance means that social workers must constantly ask the question 'What aspect of language, religion, "race" and culture matter to whom and in connection with what issues?' Sometimes these are things of primary importance to personal or group identity, sometimes they are secondary to other matters such as efficiency or speed of action. The best expert on what matters is the service user and carer, the best expert on making them aware that these aspects might matter, and that they should be taken very seriously, is the social worker.

Trying to do all this through the medium of words is exceedingly difficult, although much can and must be achieved by careful use of language and communication. Allowing flexibility of action, and seeing what matters by activities and actions, is a strong additional strand to word-based exchanges, and it is precisely in this area ('tasks') that task-centred practice has notable strengths. Perhaps because of this, alongside its deep commitment to people's views and wishes, task-centred practice has been described positively by black and minority ethnic critics of mainstream social work (Ahmad 1990).

Task-centred practice needs its practitioners to have an open and respectful view of the cultural identity of service users and carers, and as we shall see later, it provides methods to help enact this. Of course it does not solve difficulties of access to services that result from discrimination, nor is it a substitute for all of the other policies that should be in place to make sure services genuinely reflect multicultural Britain. But at the practice, rather than the policy, level it puts in place a series of values and actions that are perhaps unique in their ability to respond to the widely differing cultural backgrounds and preferences of people (Activity 1.1).

ACTIVITY 1.1: LEARNER

Reflecting back on recent learning, how were you taught about practice development?

Reflect back on some recent learning you have been doing in social work. Thinking about the knowledge base of the material you were working with, how did it involve the three elements of the practice base: research, user views and preferences, and practitioner experience? Was one given precedence over the other, was that right? Was none of these very prominent? Would you describe the learning as leading to professional practice which can and should adapt to different circumstances, or do you think it was designed to lead to routinised practice which does not adapt much? What opportunities and challenges do you think there are for you to develop professional practice in the light of your analysis?

TASK-CENTRED PRACTICE

Task-centred social work has its origins in the pioneering work of William (Bill) Reid. His contribution to practice development in social work has been immense. From the very earliest days, through over forty years of studies, he has developed practice-based research; starting his work in a practice problem, and producing material which practitioners could directly use. Along with other colleagues he has built the evidence for task-centred practice.

In the early 1960s Bill Reid's doctoral thesis (Reid 1963) looked at the influence of training and experience on judgements that social workers made about different cases. From this earliest stage his work was founded on direct empirical studies, and it was also concerned with implementation issues. Both of these strands can be seen throughout the development of task-centred work.

Reid continued his studies into social work practice, working with Ann Shyne, and delivering much of the outline of task-centred practice that was to be developed over the coming years, in a study they published as *Brief and Extended Casework* (Reid and Shyne 1969). The study built on work that had shown, counter-intuitively, that shorter periods of work could be as productive as longer ones, and began to explore why this might be. Most people would expect longer service to have a greater impact than shorter service, and in many circumstances this might be the case. But in dealing with the sort of problems brought to social workers this did not appear to be the case. Longer was not always better. If this was the case could it be capitalised on by work being broken down into small constituent parts, and then the resulting series of short-term projects should produce the maximum gain. This was exactly what was proposed, and building within the social work value base, and always working within the world of social work (as compared with other practice models beginning and being based in psychology or psychotherapy) the task-centred model has been constructed.

How can people be helped to understand the component parts of the problems they face when users so often say that they are overwhelming? How can people's strengths be used in the context of seeking help? How can the small projects, which came to be called tasks, be best used, and what methods help with their creation? These and other questions lie behind the construction of task-centred social work. Many researchers, and hundreds of postgraduate students working on their own PhDs or Masters degrees, have built a knowledge base to answer these questions.

The research evidence base has been built alongside that derived from service users and from practitioners.

Task-centred work has service user views at its core. As we have mentioned, there are reasons to do this that can be based firmly on research (Marsh and Fisher 1992) and on the values of working for, not on, service users and carers (General Social Care Council 2002). From the very start of the work the expressed views and preferences of people are central. Finding ways to help people express them as clearly as possible is a prime practitioner task. The tasks that are developed help to explore the views, they provide another way of articulating them alongside language or writing. They allow for a demonstration of views by doing. Practitioners do not seek to interpret these views and then act on them, although they may at times challenge them, and of course they will need to put them on one side if they are abusive or illegal. The service user's views, with suitable caveats about abuse, ethics and the law, are consistently driving the work of a task-centred practitioner.

Practitioner development has also played a key role, greatly aided by the fact that task-centred work has a terminology that is used to describe its different elements. For example, tasks have a definition and a technical meaning; you cannot call any action undertaken as part of the work a task. This sharing of meaning allows practitioners to share their work, and the capability of describing the work allows for practitioner development of it. For an individual practitioner it allows them to draw on their experience in a cumulative way, it allows them to build up their own knowledge as they can categorise it, and see its application. For a group of practitioners it allows for a discussion to have a common base. As we have noted earlier there is no need for translation.

The argument so far has been that social work relies on knowledge that may be based on a variety of different disciplines, but that the central dilemma for social workers is applying that knowledge. Social workers need to apply the knowledge in the complex situations of legal frames, of the varied views of people, and often in connection with problems that are particularly knotty, where the parties to these problems appear 'stuck' and where solutions are thin on the ground.

Social work needs to use evidence from research, the experience of practitioners and the views of service users and carers to develop its applied practice. It needs an open and respectful stance to the legitimate views and diverse lifestyles of people. It needs to respect diversity, and find a way to work appropriately within the varying views, cultures and ethnic origins of the people it serves. Social workers cannot do this by learning all about every aspect of these views, cultures and ethnic origins. Although they should have some broad relevant knowledge of the main strands of the societies they work in, the fact is that the real experts on these issues of cultural competence are the service users and carers themselves. Can a model for practice be developed which has this at its heart, and yet still manages to be suitable for the wide range of legal issues in social work, and to build on research, and provide a language that allows practitioners to develop their experience in a cumulative fashion (Activity 1.2)?

ACTIVITY 1.2: SUPERVISOR

Underpinning knowledge

How are you building your learning on the different strands that underpin task-centred practice? What systems do you use to search, appraise and store the following:

- legal knowledge
- research knowledge
- service user and carer views and experiences
- practice-based knowledge.

Do these areas all represent the same challenges to you regarding search, appraise and store?

There is an example answer in the Appendix.

THE TASK-CENTRED MODEL

As a model of applied practice, task-centred work is like the job itself: relatively simple to describe and relatively complex to do. It draws on the elements we have been describing so far to provide a sequence of actions based on engaging the skills, knowledge and understanding of service users and carers. An outline is given below of the key components and each one of these is covered in more detail in Chapter 2.

Mandate

Underpinning all of the work is the central question of 'What mandate do you have to undertake your work?' Social work is an activity that touches the heart of people's lives: things are revealed to social workers that are often very private, personal and emotional. To hear and to help is a privilege, based either on the person's willingness to do this because of seeking help or because there is no choice given the law.

These two elements, the informed consent of the service user, or the requirements of the law, are the twin potential mandates for a task-centred social worker.

Problems and goals

People come to social workers because they believe they have social problems, or because others, via the court, are forcing them to address social problems. Something is wrong.

Within the things that are wrong, the people, or the court, will have some idea of what is wanted. The things that are wanted are going to be the goals of any intervention.

These two elements, things that are wrong and things that are wanted form the twin focus for task-centred social work.

'Problems' are things that are wrong, and 'goals' are things that are wanted.

As we will see the goal is not necessarily, indeed is probably rarely, a complete solution to the problem. Finding out about problems will help to find the right goal, and finding the right goal will help the overall chance of success.

Goals

The point of the task-centred work is to reach the goal or goals. They are the objectives of the work, shared between service user and carer and the social worker. As the purpose of the work they provide the key measure of success.

Goals need to be directly relevant to the world of the service user and carer. Expressing the goals requires some complex activities (for example making goals specific rather than loose) but the expression also needs to reflect the emphasis in task-centred work on the relevance of the problems and goals to the world of the service user and carer. Using people's own words to express goals will be an important way of making sure that they are relevant.

Exploring problems

We have deliberately mentioned goals before problems, because they are central to the success of the work. Problems will, however, be the main issue on people's minds when they meet social workers. Moving from the expression of the problem ('what is wrong') to the expression of the goal ('what is wanted') is an important focus of the first stages of task-centred work.

Exploration of problems needs to make sure that people move beyond the immediate issues that they are worried about (or that a court requires them to worry about). These issues can be strongly directed by views of the 'right' things for social workers to deal with (for example that social workers help with the care of children, but not access to welfare rights), or by prejudice that people have encountered in the past which makes them reluctant to mention certain areas (for example the experience of racism from past services).

Social workers need to be sensitive to the range of issues that may not be immediately brought to light, as they explore initial problem stories.

Focusing problems

Social work does not usually deal with the straightforward problem. Typically people will have complex and interrelated problems, and these will be relatively long standing. Providing a means of assessing which problems are a priority for people, and linking them to any priorities enforced by legal processes, is crucial to successful problem-solving. Naming and organising problems, then putting them in priority, is part of the foundation for task-centred work. At the same time, and again a complex skill, there is a need to explore what steps have been taken to deal with these problems, to avoid repeating failures, and to build on any strengths that these steps reveal.

Refining goals

Goals, like problems, will need careful work to assess priorities, and to make them realistic and clear. Moving from general problems to more specific problems, to priority problems, has its parallel in moving from more general goals, usually expressed in people's own words, to more specific goals that will sometimes sound more technical in their language. Goals will form the measure of success of the work: a constant check for the service user and carer and for the worker as to how things are doing, and how much the work is on the right track.

Time limits

As we have seen, task-centred work is based in part on the finding that shorter periods of work can have as much impact as longer ones. Time limits can make work more productive. Motivation tends to increase as deadlines approach. They also provide a means for all parties to the work to assess priorities, and to continue to reflect on whether appropriate progress is being made.

The recorded agreement

Mandates, problems, goals and time limits will play crucial roles in the lives of service users and carers. They need to be recorded. Finding a means to provide this record may need to cope with literacy problems, and will always need to be sympathetic to the views, circumstances and uniqueness of each service user and carer.

Things that are of great importance in our lives will always have some form of record. The recorded agreement reflects the importance of the foundations of mandates, problems, goals and time limits.

Tasks and the task role

Tasks provide the incremental changes on the path from selected priority problem(s) to selected priority goal(s). They are the engine of change. Tasks do things of direct relevance to achieving the goal. They are always part of an overall plan.

They are activities undertaken by social workers, and by service users and carers. They may involve work together, they may involve co-ordinated work, they may need rehearsal or support.

Tasks are not intentions; tasks are actions. The commitment to them is a serious one for all parties.

Tasks, as we have argued, are the ways that the complex and unique situations of different people can be addressed, and they are the heart of the task-centred work.

Task development

Developing tasks is difficult. There is a balance to be struck between the democratic aim of providing full participation, and the need to use the expertise of the service user and carer or social worker as appropriate. Once a task is developed, then questions like 'is it fully understood, are there obstacles in its path, are there rehearsal or support elements needed?' are required. A great deal is now known about the broad kinds of tasks that may be suitable for some goals and problems (see, for example, Reid 2000) and about the best ways to help task development, but the details of tasks will always be unique to any one situation, and to any one individual or family or group identity. Tasks are the bridge into the world of the particular service user and carer.

Review

Predicting exactly the effectiveness of a task is hard. Making other parts of life 'stand still' while tasks on this part of it are carried out is impossible. Problems change, goals may be refined. For many reasons it is important that progress is reviewed in task-centred work. Review of problems, of goals and in particular of tasks, guides the work throughout.

Ending and evaluating

Task-centred work is time limited. There is a planned ending. The review at that point is effectively an evaluation of the overall work. If things have worked reasonably well then new skills will have been learned, and some success in the movement to the goal(s) will be evident. Neither ending nor overall evaluation are a surprise.

Continuing

The need for a time limit does not of course rule out the possibility of extension, nor of work that is composed of a series of time limits. Indeed a number of circumstances of continuing care may indicate the need for a rolling programme of time-limited agreements. But extension is never assumed, it is negotiated and purposeful, and the need for continuing agreements does not reduce the value of the time limit of the current one.

TASK-CENTRED WORK IN VARIED SETTINGS

The task-centred development work has been carried out in a wide variety of settings with a wide variety of service users and carers. Studies have covered work with children and families (Butler *et al.* 1978; Tolson and Reid 1981; Fortune 1985) and with older people (Dierking *et al.* 1980; Rathbone-McCuan 1985; Naleppa and Reid 1998). They have also covered specialities, such as mental health (Brown 1977; Gibbons *et al.* 1978 1984), foster care and adoption (Rooney 1981; Rzepnicki 1982), probation (Goldberg *et al.* 1984b) and juvenile justice (Larsen and Mitchell 1980). The model has been developed and tested in group work (Garvin 1985; Macy-Lewis 1985), with families and communities (Tolson *et al.* 1994), and in specific work areas such as social work with involuntary service users (Marsh and Fisher 1992; Rooney 1992), supervision of students (Rooney 1988; Caspi and Reid 2002) and management (Parihar 1984). Task-centred work's strength has been developed and demonstrated throughout the different specialisms in social work.

DEVELOPING TASK-CENTRED PRACTICE: THE CHALLENGE

This development has taken place within a confusing situation for the use of theory in practice in social work. First, as we have already noted, practice development is an undervalued activity within social work. Second, despite, or possibly because of this, there are potentially a bewildering number of theoretical approaches to practice that have been outlined, to a greater or lesser extent, as social work practice methods or theories. Again, as noted earlier, the *Blackwell Encyclopaedia of Social Work* lists 106 'methods' and 42 'theories' (Davies 2000). In a major national study of UK social work education, covering over 700 respondents it was found that newly qualified staff identified over 80 theorists or theoretical approaches to social work (Marsh and Triseliotis 1996: 51). Within this the top two were 'counselling' at 15 per cent and task-centred social work at 14 per cent.

Third, the same study noted the desire to continue with the application of theory (around 80 per cent said that they often or sometimes tried to apply theoretical approaches to their practice), but also the lack of support to do this (it was reported that 60 per cent of supervision sessions hardly ever or never mentioned the application of theory) (see Activity 1.3).

ACTIVITY 1.3: PRACTITIONER

Using supervision to develop practice

Before your next supervision session, conduct a quick review of your recent work to see how far you have incorporated:

- research-based evidence
- user views and preferences
- practice experience.

Share this review with your supervisor and consider how you might best develop the three areas in the future.

So the context for the development of task-centred practice is a difficult one, with a low profile generally for practice theory, and low support for it. In such a situation it is probably most sensible to see the practice of a particular model of practice, and its development and support, as something that is likely to be new to the individual, and new to the organisation. Despite its impressive pedigree, task-centred practice is an 'innovation' in social work (Box 1.3).

BOX 1.3: INNOVATION

An innovation is an idea, practice, or object that is perceived as new by an individual or other unit of adoption. It matters little, so far as human behaviour is concerned, whether or not the idea is objectively new as measured by the lapse of time since its first use or discovery. The perceived newness of the idea for the individual determines his or her reaction to it. If the idea seems new to the individual, it is an innovation.

(Rogers 1995: 11)

For many staff and for many organisations, the term 'task-centred' work will not be novel, but the detail of the model, and the skills and knowledge that are needed to enact and support it will be new. Introducing or supporting this innovation will be a difficult task. In a study conducted within a number of different social services organisations, over a substantial period of time, Gerry Smale examined many of the common methods of introducing such innovations (Smale 1998). Many of these methods appeared either weak, or in practice to be counterproductive. Indeed Smale and his colleagues were surprised to find that the most common methods seemed to act in a way that inoculated the organisation against the innovation. In a paradoxical manner the attempt to introduce the change built up the organisation's resistance to that change (see Box 1.4).

BOX 1.4: INOCULATION AGAINST INNOVATION

Many common methods of change actually work to inoculate an organisation against innovation, according to Smale (1996). They do not promote real change, they STALL. The following are the main stalling mechanisms of change.

STALL

- *Set up a pilot project to debug your innovation*
  This buys time, and enables you either to evaluate before the innovation could prove effective, or to wait for results until the innovation is obsolete. The main advantage, however, is that it enables the bulk of the organisation to work out why the innovation cannot be adopted by them.
- *Tell them to change in writing*
  Draft new guidelines/procedures/instructions. You demonstrate that you have adopted the innovation and that failure is their fault, or the innovation's, or both. You are protected from criticisms and it is rarely enough to get them to change their practice even if they want to; change what you say but not what you do.
- *Add thc innovation to custom and practice*
  Do not introduce new resources, but even if you do they are likely to be absorbed by the status quo unless you stop old practices.
- *Leave dissemination to natural forces*
  Either through the formal channels of communication down the hierarchy or the logic of the innovation's advantages, keep training short and based on individuals; don't give staff time to exchange ideas.
- *Lead through reorganisation*
  This also buys considerable time. It has the added advantages of providing you with the opportunity of getting rid of difficult staff and giving the others an example of what could happen to them if they forget who is the boss.

(Smale 1996: 36–27)

While other chapters in this book will provide many solutions for introducing, learning, supporting and developing task-centred practice it is important at this stage to be clear about the level of challenge that is being faced. Smale's work has indicated that many popular and traditional methods, such as pilot projects, new guidelines, adding on changes, low key dissemination and structural reorganisation, can, in practice, make it more difficult to introduce innovations. All of these elements are relatively common in social services: it is not easy introducing innovation in applied practice (see Activity 1.4).

ACTIVITY 1.4: TRAINER

How can training help to overcome the STALL logic?

Look at each of the elements of Box 1.4. Consider a number of recent training sessions and programmes you have run. How far have they faced problems to do with STALL? How might this be addressed in future programmes?

DEVELOPING TASK-CENTRED PRACTICE: THE OPPORTUNITY

While we must recognise the challenge of introducing task-centred practice, we should also note the substantial opportunity that this particular model offers for successful innovation. In later chapters we will be introducing a wide range of ideas that work well with task-centred work and that have proved successful in introducing this 'innovation'. But we should also note that task-centred development, because of its particular characteristics, may be reasonably cost-effective to establish within social work.

First, there is evidence from Stocking's work on the diffusion of innovations. This suggests that innovations which fit in reasonably well with existing 'climates of opinion' and 'roles of staff' may diffuse quite rapidly if suitably promoted (Stocking 1985: 80). We have already discussed the strong connection of task-centred work with two key 'climates of opinion' around evidence-based practice, and the promotion of partnership with service users and carers. We have also seen that it fits well with social work roles via its developmental base within social work itself. Stocking's research would suggest a good likelihood of relatively rapid diffusion if new approaches to development, avoiding the pitfalls noted earlier in this chapter, can establish a reasonable base for task-centred practice.

Second, there is a substantial role for service users and carers in the development of task-centred practice. As a model that emphasises partnership, and that has proved itself effective, service users and carers are likely to welcome its more widespread use. But also its underpinning principles of development emphasise the key role that people play, and this will be a major strength in the context of the growing role of service users and carers in service review, priority and management (Turner and Evans 2004) (see Activity 1.5).

ACTIVITY 1.5: SERVICE USER AND CARER

Helping social services learn: developing task-centred practice

- How can you best help social work services learn about good practice?
- What three messages would you give to social work services about taking people who use the services seriously?

Third, managers may also see a major opportunity in the development of task-centred practice, because of its strong base within mainstream social work and its application in such a wide range of service settings. Task-centred practice can take its place within a full range of services; it is not a specialised add on. There will be no need to reinvent the approach for the reality of modern-day social work, and it has proved itself flexible enough to cover a wide variety of specialised settings. The need for adaptation, either to the 'real world' of social work, or to the creation of new specialisms as services evolve, should be substantially lower with task-centred practice (Activity 1.6).

ACTIVITY 1.6: MANAGER

How difficult will it be to develop task-centred work?

Using some careful observation of behaviour and practices (see ideas in Kearney 1998), consider the following questions (derived from Smale 1996: 36–37) regarding the introduction of task-centred work. They will help to encourage change and show the degree of change that is or is not required

What changes and what stays the same?

For people

- For whom is the status quo a problem?
- Who wants change and for what reasons?
- How do the service users or customers see the problem?

For the organisation

- What changes are required to tackle the problem?
- What are the innovations involved in the proposed changes?
- Can they be changed to fit local circumstances?
- What needs to change?
- What can and should stay the same?

KEY POINTS

- ☐ Social work practice involves issues of power and control, and often complex and conflicting views: models of practice must address these issues and views.
- ☐ Practice knowledge should be based on the evidence from research, practice experience, and service user and carer experience and wishes.
- ☐ Models of practice in social work need to enable an open and respectful view of the cultural identity of service users and carers, and provide methods to enact this.
- ☐ Task-centred practice derives from work within social work, and addresses the key areas required of a social work practice model.
- ☐ Developing practice requires an understanding of why attempts at innovation often result in little real change.

KEY READING

Marsh, P. and Fisher, M. (1992) *Good Intentions: Developing Partnership in Social Services* York: Joseph Rowntree Foundation

This project introduces partnership-based social work, showing both the obstacles and the opportunities of this way of working.

Smale, G. (1996) *Mapping Change and Innovation* London: HMSO

Smale's analysis of the ways that change can be achieved includes practical guidance to help make it most likely that attempts at change will lead to positive outcomes.

Trinder, L. and Reynolds, S. (eds) (2000) *Evidence-based Practice: A Critical Appraisal* Oxford: Blackwell Science

The chapters outline the key issues in the development of evidence-based practice, and provides examples from social work and other related areas.

CHAPTER 2

STUDY

OBJECTIVES

By the end of this chapter you should:

- Recognise key issues in the choice of a method of social work
- Understand the structure of the model of task-centred social work
- Be able to analyse the nature of the mandate in social work practice
- Be able to distinguish clearly between problems and goals
- Understand the role of tasks and of review within task-centred practice.

STUDYING TASK-CENTRED PRACTICE: AN OUTLINE OF A MODEL

For many decades there have been books and articles describing social work 'methods'. Task-centred social work will usually feature as one of those methods.

A social work practice method has a set of boundaries that define it. First, it is systematic, it has a coherence, it works as an entity. Second, it will have connections to one or more particular bodies of knowledge, perhaps organised into a theory or theories. Third, it will have been tested in social work settings with social work issues. Fourth, it will need to be explicit about its value base, clear about the ethical dimensions connected with its prescriptions. Last, it will need to have an associated technology, telling us how to use it in practice: this cannot just be an exhortation, it does need to provide clear advice (see Box 4.2).

But even a brief outline of task-centred work indicates that there are a number of 'methods' contained within the task-centred system. There is a method that will establish a mandate for work, there is a method that will help to explore and select problems, there are a number of methods for different aspects of task work, and so on. If the usage was not so well established, it would be better to describe task-centred work as a set of interconnected methods. When we need to refer to this overall system we generally use the term task-centred 'model'. The task-centred model is a unified and coherent collection of methods. We will quite often refer to the model in this sense. Much of what we now describe, explore and analyse in this chapter will be the model, we will go into more detail about method as the book progresses.

HOW DO WE CHOOSE BETWEEN DIFFERENT MODELS?

Social workers need to choose among the range of models and methods available. This choice cannot be avoided. Professional practice is a systematic, knowledge-based activity, applying ethical standards, via relevant practice skills. Doing this activity involves using a method. Doing so involves making a choice.

How is this choice to be made? Making the choice involves making decisions as to what it should be based on. Unless we can clearly articulate the reasons for the choice we run the risk of others choosing for us, and of that choice not being based on issues of relevance to the social work task. People deserve a service that is based on clear choice of method, with clear reasons for that choice, as illustrated in the following six questions.

Do its values fit the underpinning value base of social work?

The starting point for the choice must be the underpinning value base of social work. All practice methods must address this. The English system provides a clear statement of the value base via its social work registration body, the General Social Care Council (GSCC). This Council, with a majority of service users and carers, has established a code of practice for social work that all UK social workers must endorse and actively promote (see Box 2.1). This is the bedrock of our choice of method.

We need to be sure that our method will support these principles. Task-centred work is clearly committed to each one (see Activity 2.1).

ACTIVITY 2.1: SERVICE USER AND CARER

Is the code of practice being followed?

Box 2.1 provides the code of practice headings that social workers must follow. What activities and attitudes might show that social workers were following this code in their work with you, and what might show that they were not? Sharing and discussing these with the social worker should help develop a service that is compatible with task-centred practice.

BOX 2.1: THE GENERAL SOCIAL CARE COUNCIL CODE OF PRACTICE FOR SOCIAL WORK

- Protect the rights and promote the interests of service users and carers.
- Strive to establish and maintain the trust and confidence of service users and carers.
- Promote the independence of service users while protecting them as far as possible from danger or harm.
- Respect the rights of service users while seeking to ensure that their behaviour does not harm themselves or other people.
- Uphold public trust and confidence in social care services.
- Be accountable for the quality of their work and take responsibility for maintaining and improving their knowledge and skills.

(General Social Care Council 2002)

Is it effective?

The effectiveness of a given method must also weigh in our choice. Does the given approach do what it aims to do? People have the right to a service that is most likely to produce the results that are agreed. There will always be disputes about effectiveness, and there will always be areas where it will be difficult to make a judgement about effectiveness, but an important part of choosing a method will always involve asking the question 'is it effective?'.

Task-centred work has a healthy track record of effectiveness, in many different studies, in many different areas. It combines evidence of effectiveness with an approach that takes the issue very seriously, and this combination gives it a strong claim to be a model of choice at present, and in the future.

Is it well liked?

A number of factors will affect whether or not people like a given practice method. People generally like to be respected and listened to, they respond to courtesy, to some humour when appropriate, and to seriousness when that is appropriate. These issues matter, they reflect underlying values of a method of practice, regarding its desire to take people's views seriously, and they reflect the ability of a method to tailor itself to particular situations. They also of course reflect the individual skills of a practitioner, which may be applied in all sorts of different circumstances. Because of the complex mix of the personal and the methodical in social work encounters we should be cautious about how much 'liking' a method is a dominant factor in the choice of that method, but any approach to practice that takes people seriously should certainly take 'liking' into account. Indeed, social work requires such a degree of personal collaboration between people, and often such a degree of trust around very personal matters, that 'liking' may be an important factor in effectiveness. Task-centred work comes through well on this criterion, with reports by all service users and carers that they generally like the approach and the model.

Does it fit existing needs?

Social work, we have suggested, takes place within a complex web of health, education and other services, in situations that involve intense human interactions, where there are often legal requirements, and usually complex social circumstances. A method of practice needs to fit this social work world, the method needs to fit the reality of the practice setting, and not be something that has to be shoehorned. Perhaps it can only fully do that if it is developed within social work itself. Task-centred work meets this requirement. A method with some overlaps with task-centred work, the solution-focused approach (Pichot and Dolan 2003) indicates the importance of this base within social work itself. Solution-focused work is based on a respectful stance towards people, and has some research which supports its effectiveness (Gingerich and Eisengart 2000). However, its development has been strongly based within schools, and its approach is lower on action and stronger on talk when compared with task-centred work. Ideas and developments from each method will rightly inform the other, but at present the task-centred work is clearly more applicable in social work situations, where there are often elements of compulsion, and where there is great value in a practice method that puts such a strong priority on action as part of problem exploration and solution.

Is it efficient?

All health, education and social care services have high demands on fixed budgets, and they need to make the best use of the money available. Equally, service users and carers have 'high demands on fixed budgets', sometimes budgets that are indeed financial ones, but nearly always budgets that involve substantial uses of their time and of their emotions and efforts. Working in a way that is as efficient as possible is in everyone's interests. Task-centred work tries to do this in a number of different ways. It helps with sorting out whether there are substantial grounds for doing work, it helps prioritise, it works to time limits, and it aims to leave people with more skills and resources than they started with, to help them solve future similar problems with perhaps less external input. Efficiency is important for the task-centred method.

Can it develop?

Services develop over the years, legislation changes, social demands alter; the work of a social worker is going to change as knowledge develops, and as societies make new demands, and present new opportunities. Change will always be part of an occupation like social work which is so bound up with the way that individuals, families and groups interact with society and its structures. Methods of practice must be able to reflect these changes, and build positively on them. The idea of development needs to be integral to the method of practice, so that change is a natural part of the method, not something imposed on it. In common with the emphasis on effectiveness, this process of development is built into the task-centred method (see Activity 2.2).

ACTIVITY 2.2: MANAGER

Questions regarding the choice of practice model

Consider the six questions that we have suggested should be answered regarding choice of practice model:

- Do its values fit the underpinning value base of social work?
- Is it effective?
- Is it well liked?
- Does it fit existing needs?
- Is it efficient?
- Can it develop?

How is the development of practice in your agency addressing these questions?

TASK-CENTRED PRACTICE

As we outline later, in Chapter 4, *The Task-Centred Book* is based on two decades of experience in helping practitioners to use, and to develop, the task-centred model. The work that is outlined below comes from training programmes we have run as part of this work. The two examples are chosen to show some of the variety within social work practice, where a mix of reluctance, and learning, communication and developmental challenges may well be part of the experience of service users and carers.

The two practitioners, Friyana and Kathy, worked in specialised agencies, Friyana in a child care team and Kathy in an adult service. Both the examples outlined were people who had some substantial experience of being helped by social work, but where past methods had not been as productive as desired.

The first example is Louise (all names and identifiable circumstances have been changed), where there were difficulties in parenting, as outlined in Box 2.2.

The second example is Dave, who has not been well cared for in his childhood, and whose ability to care for himself is somewhat limited by this and by developmental and learning difficultics (scc Box 2.3 and Activity 2.3).

ACTIVITY 2.3: TRAINER

Developing a stock of examples from existing practice

The use of examples from existing practice is a powerful way of making sure that training does really address practice issues and helps practice to develop. How might you develop a 'stock' of these examples, for instance by the direct involvement of practitioners in training, by the use of portfolio materials and so on?

BOX 2.2: LOUISE, A SERVICE USER

Louise was referred to specialist child care services for work on her parenting skills.

Louise's 4-year-old daughter was recently freed for adoption. Her son Steven is 2 years old, subject to a full Care Order and on the Child Protection Register (category: neglect – lifestyle of carer). Steven lives with Louise at present. Main concerns have been:

- failure to thrive (intensive work from paediatrician, dietician and health visitor)
- safety in home
- anonymous allegations that Louise leaves Steven alone in the home or with unsuitable people.

Louise wishes to work towards having the Care Order discharged. As part of this work the community team social worker referred her to me for

- assessment of parenting skills
- work to develop parenting skills.

(Portfolio H 1996: 2.1)

BOX 2.3: DAVE, A SERVICE USER

Dave was referred to the Community Adult Team for support to move out into the community to live independently.

Dave's family has been involved with social workers since he was a baby. His mother had problems with relationships with her first husband and subsequent partners, and her parenting skills were poor. Although help and advice was offered, the family unit could not be maintained as a whole and Dave and his siblings were split up and placed in care.

Dave has mild learning difficulties and during his school life he was bullied and very unhappy.

His grandmother helped to bring Dave up, but most of the time his mother intervened and he was placed back into foster care.

The only sibling Dave is close to is his sister Sheila and in recent years they have been reunited and become close.

At present Dave is staying with Sheila, but this is only a temporary arrangement. Sheila is a single mother with two young boys who have been diagnosed with Fragile X syndrome, which is a chromosome disorder causing varying degrees of learning difficulty and associated behavioural problems.

Sheila can see in Dave some of the traits she sees in her two sons and has, with the agreement of Dave, seen his GP and a test for Fragile X is to be carried out in the near future.

Dave is very much a loner and has no close friends. His sister Sheila is concerned that if Dave gets a flat and lives independently, he will be vulnerable and need support. She will be moving to Scotland shortly, when support for Dave will be even more important.

(Portfolio E 2000: 2.1)

MODEL STRUCTURE

The overall process in task-centred work is to build from a firm mandate for the work, via prioritised problems, to agreed goals within a set time period. The work does this by using a set of activities, agreed at regular intervals by practitioner and service users and carers, which build towards the final goals. Each of the activities, known as tasks, requires careful development and review. The process of review is fundamental to the work, encouraging assessment of direction, progress, accountability and motivation during the work, and also assessing eventual outcome at the end point.

This structure is relatively simple to explain, but often much harder to enact. The process is designed to be transparent to everyone involved and at an early stage of the work it is important that the model is briefly outlined. Each party to the work should, ideally, always understand what they are doing and why.

The explanation does not have to be very detailed. One person summed up the model themselves, after the practitioner attempted an explanation, in a very succinct fashion, by likening it to a set of steps, where the treads are the review of the work and the risers are the tasks leading to the goal or goals (Portfolio K 2002: 5.3D) (see Box 2.4).

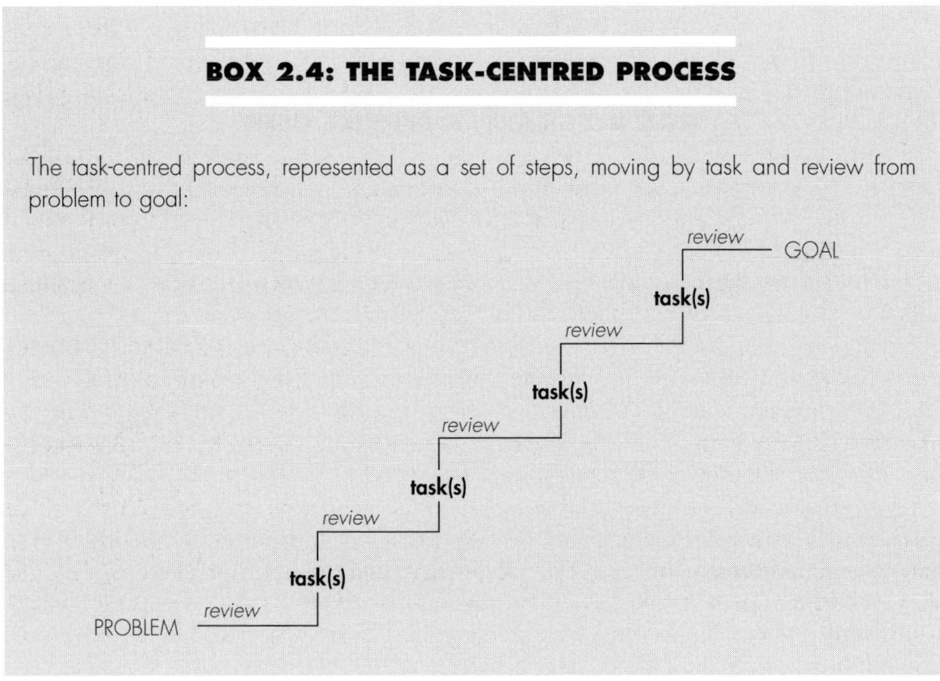

BOX 2.4: THE TASK-CENTRED PROCESS

The task-centred process, represented as a set of steps, moving by task and review from problem to goal:

The introduction of the model is part of the overall process of working in partnership. This partnership must be based on a common understanding of the reasons for doing the work. This mandate for the work underpins all that follows.

Mandate

The basic principle underlying task-centred work is that there are two fundamental reasons why social workers, service users and carers undertake work together. One derives from the expressed wishes of people, the other from the fact that there is a legal requirement to undertake the work, even if it has not been requested.

Neither of these reasons is likely, in the real world of social work, to be totally straightforward.

The 'expressed wishes' of service users and carers, for example, may be in part motivated by pressure from others. The important issue for task-centred work is that, on balance, these are genuine wishes and that the option of saying, 'No thank you, I don't want the service' has been seriously considered and rejected. It is probably common for there to be ambivalence when requesting a service of any sort, so there is room for some doubt in this mandate, but there should be a clear recognition that its base is a voluntary agreement.

On the other hand the second reason, the legal requirement for the work, has an element of compulsion. For example, the issue of the care of a child or of an older person, may need to be raised whether the person wishes it to be raised or not. For this mandate the option of 'no service thank you' is not available. In task-centred work, as in all methods of social work, the practitioner should work hard to make it very clear exactly why the issue is being raised, and what the legal requirements are to raise it. Dependent on the nature of the legal requirement there will be a certain level of continuing involvement irrespective of a person's wishes, until a judgement can be made, via appropriate legal mechanisms, that there is no continuing compulsory need for involvement.

This underlying compulsion may or may not lead to the possibility of task-centred practice. The complete rejection of the mandate by the service user and carer could make it impossible to carry out task-centred work. If there is a complete rejection of the legal requirement, a denial for example, that there is any problem at all despite a court hearing and an order, then it will not be possible to engage in task-centred work. Under these circumstances some form of 'social policing' will need to be undertaken.

Task-centred work is based on one, or both, of these twin mandates. Either the expressed wishes of the service user and carer, or the agreement, however reluctant, that there is a legal requirement for the work to be done. Of course both mandates can be present. There can be a compulsory element of the work, accompanied by a freely entered into agreement to work on some other area.

Task-centred work does highlight, via the process of exploring the mandate, where agreement is not possible, and where either service may not continue or 'social policing' may be required because of refusal to accept legal requirements. In either case the door should be held open for a return to task-centred practice. In 'voluntary' situations this will be the possibility of future contact, and encouragement to make this contact if circumstances change. In 'compulsory' situations there will have to be continuing contact, but regular attempts will need to be made to see if the agreement could be renegotiated so that the legal basis is accepted and there can be a shared development of work on this basis.

This approach to the mandate rules out one area of work for the task-centred practitioner. Task-centred practice will not take place where the practitioner believes there to be a problem, but where the service user and carer do not, and where there is no legal requirement to help with or control the problem. If, following serious discussion where all the important issues that the practitioner thinks should be raised have been raised, a person says they do not want the service, then that is the end, unless the law insists otherwise.

The approach, in common with others, also leaves a number of areas where the issue of a 'legal requirement' will be a difficult judgement to make. Child protection work, for example, often has a professional decision-making system that leads to a professional judgement that involvement should be maintained irrespective of a person's wishes. Child protection conferences, following investigations that are based on the law, could come to such views. These professional but court-like decision-making bodies will often raise mandate problems for practitioners, service users and carers alike. Task-centred work does not make these problems more difficult, nor any easier, but it does highlight the fine border line between compulsion and voluntarism that there can be in parts of social work. Task-centred practitioners will do their best to move the mandate towards clear bases in expressed wishes or legal requirement, and this may be a continuing part of the work.

Friyana faced this difficulty in the work with Louise (Portfolio H 1996: 2.2). She was clear there were grounds for involvement that Louise accepted:

> At the time of accepting this referral, the Department had a statutory mandate to work with Louise since her child Steven was living at home under a Care Order.
>
> (Portfolio H 1996: 2.2)

However, she was less sure about the work that was mandated to be done under that Care Order:

> I felt the mandate for work with Louise was a bit 'fuzzy'. While Louise had the motivation to co-operate with our Department in order to work towards getting the Care Order discharged, I was not sure to what extent she would agree with the problems as identified in the referral.
>
> (Portfolio H 1996: 2.2)

Louise also felt that there were questions about the mandate for work, and just what was required and what was optional, and she chose to use a solicitor to help her clarify this. Friyana was asked to submit her proposal for work to Louise's solicitor, and both parties evidently understood that there were going to be continuing issues about the mandate. Friyana worried about how this would affect the task-centred work, but she found that while there would continue to be some ambiguities there was scope for the work to commence:

> Initially I felt that her request for a written proposal of my work to be submitted to her solicitor, placed some constraints on my task-centred practice. However I attempted to word the proposal so as to leave space for negotiation around the problem areas.
>
> (Portfolio H 1996: 2.2).

She commented that she admired

> Louise's resourcefulness in using her solicitor to check that the proposed work was in her best interests, and thus redressing some of the imbalance of power. It certainly had the effect of putting me on my mettle, in terms of ensuring that my work with Louise was fair and was carried out in a spirit of partnership.
>
> (Portfolio H 1996: 6.1)

For Kathy the issues were less around the nature of the problems to be addressed, and more around who would provide the mandate, would it be Dave or his sister Sheila? Sheila may want help to support her brother, and Dave may want help in his own right to live more independently. As it turned out Dave was willing to work with her, and Sheila relatively unable to do so as she was moving some distance. But Dave's wishes, given his need for support, seemed to be unrealistic:

> I want a job, I know I can't get one but that is what I would like.
>
> I want to live on my own, at the seaside would be nice.
>
> (Portfolio E 2000: 2.3)

The practitioner needed to continue to work to refine these wishes, but they were the ones that formed the basis for the work, and she accepted that.

Problems and goals

A problem, or more likely a number of problems, will have led to the contact with the practitioner. They are the underlying reason for the work. But, assuming the mandate is established, they form the starting point not the end point of the work. The work is designed to lead to something all agree is wanted and desirable. It is designed to lead to a goal.

Problems are things that are wrong, and goals are things that are wanted. Problems are explored and analysed in order to clarify goals. Goals are unlikely to be complete solutions to problems. Following thorough discussion and negotiation they should be agreed by the practitioner if the person decides they are relevant, and if, especially for compulsory mandates, the practitioner agrees that they address the required problem. It is always difficult to know what will really relieve a problem, and the goal may seem surprising, but if it has been thought through by all involved, this 'surprising' goal may be very effective. There is plenty of time, and a number of mechanisms, for reviewing it as work progresses.

Goals

Goals are the desired and agreed outcomes of the work. Ideally they will need to be expressed in the person's own words, and certainly in as jargon-free language as possible.

Goals should ideally be relatively specific rather than 'fuzzy', they should be achievable, and sensibly related to the problem, for service user, carer and for practitioner (see Box 4.4 and Activity 4.4).

Friyana and Louise agreed two goals for the work:

- 'I want to stop Steven throwing a paddy when I say no.'
- 'I want Steven to understand he can't have everything his own way.'

Quite rightly Friyana worried about the second goal in particular:

> It was hard to help her to work the goal in such a way that was not 'fuzzy' and therefore not measurable or achievable. I did not feel very satisfied with the wording of her second goal because I thought it was not a very measurable goal and not a very realistic one in relation to a 2-year-old child. A better way of expressing it could have been, say, 'I want Steven to do as I tell him most of the time' or '. . . more often than he does now'. Louise was clear she did not

> expect or want a perfectly behaved child, just better behaviour. In spite of this 'fuzziness' I did feel that, because I had used Louise's own words, she had a good investment in achieving the goal. I felt the first goal was more clearly expressed, and that it was achievable. I felt both goals were desirable, in the sense that achieving them would help make Louise a better parent – if she had more control of Steven's behaviour she would probably develop a better relationship with him. Both goals were linked with the selected problems.
>
> (Portfolio H 1996: 3.3)

For Dave the goals were to:

- 'Identify a suitable college course and enrol on the course.'
- 'Attend an appointment with a genetic counsellor.'

Although the second goal seemed somewhat unrelated to living independently, it was related to his worries about Fragile X syndrome, and Kathy felt that his worries about this may be getting in the way of motivation for other activities, indeed in her discussions with Dave she found:

> Identifying both goals does appear to have motivated Dave to consider college and I am optimistic that a test for Fragile X, whether positive or negative, will motivate Dave. It may also assist in obtaining a different benefit for him. He was actually quite elated after this session that he had made decisions and agreed the agreement.
>
> (Portfolio E 2000: 3.3)

Exploring problems

Most people arrive at a service thinking it deals with certain areas of work, and they may well tailor what they say in the light of those expectations. Discussions may also be tense because of the emotional nature of the problems. There may be great pressure from the problems. All these reasons mean that getting into the details of problems at too early a stage is likely to be a mistake. Of course there may be an urgent issue that needs dealing with, for example the imminent disconnection of electricity, but this, in task-centred terms, would be called a pre-problem. It needs dealing with, and it should be, but after that a more considered approach is needed to finding out what matters most to people, and maybe adding things that matter because of legal requirements.

The process of problem exploration follows five broad stages. As in all other descriptions of task-centred work there will, in practice, be a movement back and forth between these stages, but in the interests of clarity we will describe them here as discrete and following in neat order. First, there needs to be a scan of all potential relevant problems. Second, there may need to be additions made to this by the worker, either as suggestions or as requirements if there is a legal mandate. Third, there needs to be some details provided about the problems. Fourth, there needs to be statements made that can summarise the problems, in the words of the service user and carer. Fifth, the problems need to be put in priority order and a selection made for action (see Box 4.3 for a summary).

As part of this process, task-centred practitioners also need to have an eye to the strengths that people have, and these may indicate ways that future tasks can help problem-solving. Exploring these strengths a little may also help to avoid the possibility of a feeling that 'there are just too many problems'. This sense, which some people may have, of being overwhelmed at this stage may also be alleviated by the process of breaking problems down into summarised statements, and putting them in priority for action. It is a difficult stage for practitioners to get right, when there is a need for thorough exploration, but also for recognising that there are underlying strengths. People will need to be reminded that these are steps which lead to the agreement on goals and they are not an end in themselves.

The first stage is the *scan* of problems. This is a brief view of all of the issues that might be relevant to work on, not going into detail. Often practitioners find the use of a flipchart sheet helpful at this stage, used for making short statements that provide a way into the problem issues. Louise, for example, had statements like these on her flipchart:

- 'It's hard to explain to Steven things that are happening in his life.'
- 'Since he's come back to live with me I'm having difficulty with him getting upset when I leave him, and him screaming at night.'
- 'I always give in to him.'

(Portfolio H 1996: 2.3)

The next stage is to review this scan and to make sure that any *additional problems* are raised. These might be ones that the practitioner is raising because of their knowledge, for example of child development. Or they might be ones that the practitioner is raising because of the legal requirements, for example concerns about the care of children that have been raised by others. Or they might come up from the service user and carer, as happened with Louise:

> At the second session I reminded Louise it was for her to identify the problems, and we looked in more detail at the problem scan. Louise introduced a further problem – Steven disobeying her and testing out her authority.
>
> (Portfolio H 1996: 2.4)

This was the second session with Louise, and there is a good deal of work in scanning and adding.

For the third stage each problem heading is worked with to provide some *details*. This will involve some greater understanding of the problems, and some quantification of them. It might involve being specific about other people's views of them, and again it will be done with an eye to potential strengths that are revealed behind the problem story.

The fourth stage will involve the practitioner in helping to get a *statement*, in the person's own words, that summarises the problem in a relatively succinct manner.

Finally, but most importantly, once all the problems have been explored in this way, they need to be put in some form of priority order and a *selection* made as to which one(s) will be worked on first. The practitioner may insist on one of them featuring at this stage because it is a legally mandated problem, but otherwise the selection is made by the person in the context of advice from the practitioner.

Focusing problems and refining goals

People typically face situations where the problems seem enormous, and where what they want seems unclear or unachievable. Task-centred practitioners work in partnership with people to help to resolve both these issues. Problems become more focused, goals become more refined. This is not to say that the scale of the problems is necessarily reduced, it may indeed be added to if there are legally mandated problems to be included as additions, but the nature of problems changes once they are clarified, acknowledged and made more specific.

Task-centred practitioners will work with people to help them to acknowledge problems explicitly, see how they might work on them, and focus them to be relatively specific. These activities are likely to be demanding intellectually and emotionally, and we will explore this further in later chapters.

The problems are a stage on the way to forming goals, and goals need to be refined to be as accurate as possible. The acronym SMART is well known, standing for

- Specific
- Measurable
- Achievable
- Realistic
- Timely.

Goals need to be as SMART as realistically possible. Practitioners need to help people reach these SMART goals, and in doing so they need to make sure they are genuinely helping, not directing. The only exception to this will be for legally mandated problems, where the practitioner must assess how far the goal will genuinely alleviate the mandated problem, their responsibility is to make sure that it does.

The importance of goals cannot be overemphasised. Getting them right is the key to the work. Providing a separate session just on refining goals may often be the ideal way to proceed in task-centred work (Activity 2.4).

ACTIVITY 2.4: SUPERVISOR

Helping to develop SMART goals

Developing SMART goals, but with suitably clear links to people's own words, is a vital skill of task-centred practice. Take some recent cases and review the 'SMARTness' and the service user and carer voice elements of the goals. How might you help practitioners to make goals 'SMARTer' and reflect better the voice of service users and carers?

Time limits

Time limits help greatly with both motivation and accountability. Everyone experiences the effect of working harder as time limits for a piece of work to be complete draw near, and social workers, as well as service users and carers, are no different in this respect from others. The experience of drawing up time limits is universal, because of the need to get something done in a certain period: we want the plumber to fix the bath tomorrow, or we need our telephone line fixed by this afternoon. Deadlines are used to keep others to account, to make sure that all parties to the process know the date something is needed by, and that they will be asked to account for work, done or not done, on that date.

As we have seen in Chapter 1, early studies which led to task-centred practice showed that short-term work could be just as effective as longer-term work. Sensible time limits for work therefore provide additional gains, around motivation and accountability, without loss of effectiveness. They also provide a convenient yardstick to measure progress, when it is known that the work is a 'quarter way through' for example, the speed, feasibility and so on can be assessed by all.

The time limit for reaching the goals is inevitably an estimate, but it is a vital part of the work. Experience shows that around six weeks to three months is the optimum period for the agreement to last. Within this period the frequency of contact will need to be specified. There is a need for regular contact, as we discuss in Chapter 3, but contact may vary from a number of sessions very close together at the start as work is defined, to more spread out sessions towards the end as the process becomes more well known to all parties.

The recorded agreement

Important events in our lives are usually recorded, and important transactions usually bring some formality to this process, a bill of sale or a contract for service. These act as a constant reminder of what is to be done, and signify the real commitment of the parties to do it. These records provide a way in which each partner to them can say, in a significant way, this is important to me, I have thought about it, and I agree to do it. The recorded agreement serves these functions in task-centred practice.

The recorded agreement marks the stages where people seeing social workers move properly into the category of service user or carer. Before this stage it would perhaps be better to refer to applicants, if they seek services, and respondents if they are subject to some form of potential legal mandate. The recorded agreement marks the point where both respondent/applicant and practitioner accept that work of a certain nature, based on certain reasons, to achieve certain purposes by a set time, will be done.

Recording can take many forms. Task-centred practitioners regularly use flipcharts in their work, and these could form the bullet points of an agreement (see Chapter 7). It is possible that an agreement could be typed up, or hand written, in more traditional A4 document style. Sensitivity about literacy is needed, in common with any other serious transactions where recorded agreements will play a part. It is possible to make the language very straightforward, indeed it should be in substantial part in people's own words. It is, of course, possible to run through the document with people, so that all words and commitments are clear, indeed this would be good practice and vital for clarity. It is also possible to be imaginative about the agreement, and perhaps use a taped record rather than a written one.

These issues of language, and of the philosophy of the agreement, were clearly of concern to Friyana in her work with Louise.

> In Louise's agreement the problems and goals are worded in Louise's own language ('paddy' rather than 'tantrum' for example). Although I felt that goals could have been worded a little more clearly, it was important that I reflected as closely as possible what Louise was saying. I feel Louise was assured that the problems and goals were genuinely her own, not imposed upon her. In this way the written agreement becomes a product of partnership, rather than a tool used by a person in authority in order to force a particular course of action.
>
> (Portfolio H 1996: 3.4)

Tasks and the task role

The mandate forms the starting point for the task-centred process. The recorded agreement provides the foundations that are essential for this to move into active work. The tasks are the actions that then drive on the work to try and meet the agreed goals within the set time period.

Tasks may be big or small, although too big or too small is likely to prove a mistake. They will come in many different shapes and sizes. The one connecting factor is that they have a common purpose: to take the work forward, via one step, to the agreed goal or goals. Everyone at work is doing activities, but 'task' in the connection of task-centred work is more than just an activity, it does not stand alone, it is part of an overall plan, and via review also contributes a substantial level of feedback about progress.

Although tasks are activities, and they are often done separately by the people involved, they should have a positive impact on the working relationship. Creating things, and working individually or jointly, to a common purpose, with people brings greater understanding of each other. Dave, in his review of the work, said that via task-centred work, 'we have got to know each other better and I can talk to you' (Portfolio E 2000: 5.3).

With Louise, tasks contributed directly to the empowering philosophy of task-centred work, when they gave her 'a sense she was doing something herself' (Portfolio H 1996: 4.7).

For Louise, as for other people experiencing task-centred practice, tasks offer a genuine, visible and effective means of empowerment.

Task development

There are many different kinds of task. The most basic distinction between tasks is between those that occur within sessions, and those that occur outside of them, forming 'homework' for both practitioner and service user and carer. Tasks conducted within sessions should be just as carefully thought through as those done between sessions.

The size of a task has already been mentioned. If tasks are too small they may be dismissed as trivial and if they are too large they may be unachievable. Finding the right size, to make some progress, but not so much that it is overwhelming, is difficult.

Tasks can be one-off, or something that will be repeated. We will have examples of both in other chapters.

Tasks may be individual (J will . . .), reciprocal (J will . . . and K will . . .), or shared (J and K will . . .). The judgement which will help decide which is best should be based on a judgement about overall movement to the goal. Which is most likely to help, which provides the best size, which engages key players, what level of support might be needed to achieve the task? There has been a great deal of work on tasks, including pulling together many years of research into a 'task planner' which provides a wide range of task planning ideas to generate tasks for different circumstances (Reid 2000) (see Activity 2.5).

ACTIVITY 2.5: PRACTITIONER

Keeping a log of problems and the tasks developed for them

When you start to develop your task-centred work, keep a log of the problems and the tasks that were developed for them. Over time you will be developing a personal task planner to remind you of the range of tasks that may be relevant, and as your work progresses and you can see which are more successful, you will be able to share some of the best ideas with other task-centred practitioners.

There is an example answer in the Appendix.

Task-centred practitioners need to ensure that tasks are the right size, that they will genuinely aid progress to goals, and that they are carried out in the right location with the right people (session or between session, one-off or recurring, individual, reciprocal or shared). They also need to ensure that everyone is clear exactly what is needed, and that they can and should do what is needed. Kathy, with Dave, for example:

> Ensured Dave knew where the bus station was and the whereabouts of the photo booth. Talked through the sequence of having a photograph taken in a booth. Reminded Dave to have £3 in one pound coins. Told him where to go if he had any difficulty. Reassured him that if he could not manage the task that we would look at other ways of obtaining the photographs.
>
> (Portfolio E 2000: 4.1)

In Chapter 3 we will provide some detail of the development of tasks, and provide details about a validated technique which is the most effective way to make sure that an agreed task is fully thought out and most likely to be successful.

This sense of organised planning, and smooth motion towards goals is of course an idealised version of real task-centred practice. Tasks will often be imperfect, and practitioners will get muddled just as much as service users and carers. The point is to have a constant attempt to make this progress, to struggle at all times in the work to see what actions will help the advance from problem, from what is wrong, to the goal, to what is needed.

They often require practitioners to stand back from taking over from people, and in that sense they continue the emphasis that the task-centred model places on empowerment. Of course practitioners should do work that they have particular skills to do, or where their support is crucial to progress, but the tendency to take over just because 'it's quicker if I do' should be resisted. Kathy found this in her work with Dave. As seen above, he needed a photograph from a photo booth, and Kathy commented: 'In the past to save time, I would have taken him for his photograph' (Portfolio E 2000: 2.6).

But this time, as a task-centred worker, she accepted Dave's request, and Dave reported afterwards that he 'felt proud when the task was completed, he did not expect to be able to do it' (Portfolio E 2000: 4.5).

Developing this task was hard work for Kathy. Dave's attention span was around fifteen minutes, and he was not used to being taken seriously, nor to planning things like this which he assumed he could not do. It was not easy for Kathy to work like this, and we will come back to this issue in detail in later chapters in the book. However, as a result of hard work by both Dave and Kathy, there was a successful result, a sense of pride, and not just a product gained but also a skill learnt.

Review

Once work is in progress it is regularly reviewed. It is important to make sure that work is on track towards the final goal or goals, and also to learn from the tasks that are done. Tasks that are successful may indicate new strengths to be built on, tasks that do not do well may indicate weaknesses that need help, or they may indicate poor task development and perhaps raise questions about the motivation to work on the particular area. This learning will only occur if review is built in to every task-centred session. It is not something that is just left to the end of the work (see Chapter 7).

All parties to task-centred work are engaging in learning, as Kathy put it: 'It has been a learning curve for both of us' (Portfolio E 2000: 5.4).

Time limits are built into the work regarding final outcomes, but they are also, of course, built into the session structure of the work. The gap between sessions forms a time limit for each of the agreed tasks to be undertaken. Each session will need to begin with a review of the tasks, and the progress being made to the goal or goals. The gaps between sessions need to be planned correctly for task work. Probably there will be weekly meetings, but at the start and at very active periods they could be more regular, and there may be a case for some fortnightly gaps at appropriate points.

Review also allows the work to be responsive to other events that will inevitably occur in people's lives. It allows a temporary diversion to deal with a particular issue that was not part of the original planning, and there may be opportunistic use of one-off tasks. Ideally this occurs as little as possible, but in practice there will nearly always be some minor diversions, and possibly major ones. These need acknowledging and a judgement made between everyone involved as to whether or not being temporarily 'blown off course' is the right thing to do, before continuing, perhaps in slightly modified form, with the agreed work.

Review allows people to reflect on what role they are playing in the work, a process which is more often done by professionals. Task-centred work is a genuine partnership, with all parties playing important roles. This was well understood by Louise, who wrote thoughtful notes about the way she was changing her views and actions in connection with her son. The social worker made this comment after one review:

> Louise's response to being asked what part she had played in tackling her difficulties demonstrated her commitment to the work. It describes a very significant change in Louise's parenting – an understanding of her son's needs and ability to meet those needs – which for me illustrates the efficacy of the task-centred model. When considered alongside Louise's record of numerous parenting assessments, a residential assessment, and the placing of her daughter for adoption, I feel this shows that a more client-centred method can succeed where others have failed.
>
> (Portfolio H 1996: 5.2)

The process of review may also feel somewhat threatening. Social workers will feel, rightly, that their work is being checked. Have they done what they said, have they done the tasks agreed for them? Service users and carers will also feel this, and the review parts of sessions will need to be handled with discretion, tact and thoughtfulness. There were times when Dave felt this in the work with Kathy, resulting in him not coming to one session (Portfolio E 2000: 4.6). Kathy took the opportunity to look carefully with Dave at the need for review as a genuine help to them both, and was careful to make sure that any part of the review process was handled gently and positively. By the end of the work Dave was in favour of the task-centred form of review, as he could 'see at a glance what he had achieved' (Portfolio E 2000: 5.4).

Ending and evaluating

Review is a form of constant evaluation, so the evaluation at the end of work is not in any sense a surprise, and in some ways is a summary of the reviews throughout. The end of the work is an opportunity to consider overall progress towards the goal, and its relation to reducing problems. It is a time to reflect on the part that is played by people in the work, and to consider the future.

Louise, for example, said the work had made a lot of difference to her. In particular she found it helpful:

- choosing two problems
- talking it over with the social worker
- having the social worker present to observe Steven's problem behaviour
- putting new skills into practice in sessions.

Louise further reported that she was now giving Steven more time and that she was more relaxed with him. Steven would now usually listen to Louise without her having to raise her voice. Most encouragingly, Louise felt their relationship was better. There had been times when she felt like giving him up and asking him to be accommodated beforehand, whereas now she looked forward to each day with him – 'even the days when he was naughty' (Portfolio H 1996: 5.3).

The work with Dave did not achieve the goal that was wanted, one that both parties to the work had agreed was very difficult to achieve at the outset. But it did achieve a very positive outcome in terms of skills and self-image via obtaining a bus pass, which itself had played a very positive role in Dave's life. Kathy highlighted the change in goal, when she commented 'it did not end as I would have wished but on reflection it has been successful' (Portfolio E 2000: 5.2).

Continuing

There will almost certainly be a partial success in reaching goals. In Dave's case a much simpler outcome was reached, but one which was very helpful to him now and in the future. The partial reaching of a goal does not mean that the work should automatically be extended. More of the same is unlikely to be sensible unless work has gone dramatically wrong because of substantial and unpredicted circumstances outside of anyone's control. If this does happen it is probably best to suspend the work, and then renegotiate it, perhaps quite briefly and start out again.

On the other hand the work could have thrown up new problems that need to be tackled, and this should be considered seriously. A new agreement may be reached.

Some aspects of social work require continuing involvement, and this will continue around the task-centred work. Contact before the agreement and contact after are quite possible, but the actual task-centred work should stand alone within this (see Activity 2.6).

ACTIVITY 2.6: LEARNER

Reviewing the elements of task-centred work

Think about the following elements: have you understood each one? Put the elements in order of difficulty as you see it, for your personal learning of the model. Why are some harder than others? How can you make sure you overcome learning the more difficult ones?

- mandate
- problems and goals
- goals
- exploring problems
- focusing problems
- refining goals
- time limits
- the recorded agreement
- tasks and the task role
- task development
- review
- ending and evaluating
- continuing.

FAMILIES AND GROUPS

Much of social work will be undertaken with families and with groups of people. It is important to be careful about the form of agreement that applies in this case. It should not automatically be assumed that one overall agreement with shared goals is the only model that can apply in these circumstances. As well as this 'group' agreement with 'group' goals there are two other forms of agreement that could be negotiated and that will be appropriate in a number, perhaps the majority, of cases. The first is to have a 'group' agreement (say with three family members), but to have different goals for each of the signatories to the agreement. This will allow the work to begin from the common problems of the group, just as in the one single agreement model, but it will reflect the different needs of different members. The second alternative to one overall agreement is to have different agreements with different members of the 'group', but with some common elements, for example some common problems, and where the overall work is linked, perhaps in time, perhaps via review, across the different agreements.

These three approaches could be summarised as the *collaboration model*, where there is one common agreement, the *co-operation model*, where there is a group agreement but with different goals for different members, and the *co-ordination model*, where there are separate agreements linked in some more general way. No one of these is necessarily superior to another, they are different solutions for different circumstances.

CHOOSING TASK-CENTRED WORK

Earlier in this book we have suggested a number of reasons why task-centred work is of great value to people in getting an efficient, effective, relevant and well-liked service. It is of value to social workers for similar reasons, and also because it can span the voluntary and compulsory aspects of the job. It can also show where a partnership way of working, such as task-centred work, is simply unachievable and where some form of social policing is the only option.

There are a few circumstances, except for those that make partnership working completely impossible, where task-centred work would not be applicable, relevant and suitable. One is where the overriding need is for personal reflection and analysis. Sometimes requests for help are about the need to mull over issues and to see the many sides that most situations have. If there is no need or desire for action then task-centred work is not needed. A second set of situations does make it extremely hard, and perhaps impossible to undertake task-centred work. It revolves around lives where the ability to exercise any degree of control seems to be next to impossible. It may be people with serious psychotic illness and at times little grasp on reality. It may be the family whose complex interlocking history of problems is generating crisis after crisis at such speed that negotiating an agreement is simply not possible. In these circumstances working towards task-centred work is the most likely option. Extreme circumstances like these will always be at the edge of professional practice knowledge, there are no easy solutions.

BUILDING A NEW PROFESSIONALISM

In this chapter, and in Chapter 1, we have shown the elements of task-centred practice, and their rationale and origins. Despite the long pedigree of task-centred work, these elements, all together, do represent a new way of working when compared with many of the models in social work and in other professions. The idea of genuine and active partnership work, reflected in openness about mandates, in joint activities, in accountability and in review, is built up in task-centred work into something which develops a new sense of the meaning of the word 'professional' (Verbeek 1997). 'Professionalism' in this model involves sharing knowledge and control of the work, and a recognition that relationships and shared experiences are very important to good outcomes (Davies 1998) (see Box 2.5).

BOX 2.5: OLD AND NEW CONCEPTS OF PROFESSIONALISM

Old professionalism

- *mastery of knowledge*: unilateral decision process (patient as dependent, colleagues as deferential)
- *autonomy and self-management*: individual accountability
- *detachment*: interchangeability of practitioners.

New professionalism

- *reflective practice*: interdependent decision process (patient as empowered, colleagues involved)
- *supported practice*: collective responsibility
- *engagement*: specificity of practitioners' strengths.

(Davies 1998: 193)

KEY POINTS

- ☐ 'Choosing a method of social work' should involve consideration of
  - ☐ its value base
  - ☐ its effectiveness
  - ☐ how well it is liked by service users and carers
  - ☐ the 'fit' to existing needs in social services
  - ☐ its efficiency
  - ☐ its capacity to develop.
- ☐ Task-centred practice is based on the expressed wishes of service users and carers and/or a legal requirement for work that is accepted by them.
- ☐ Problems are what is wrong, goals are what is wanted, and it is vital that a task-centred practitioner distinguishes the two.
- ☐ Problem exploration involves scanning, adding problems if needed, providing details, obtaining an agreed service user and carer statement, and the selection of priorities.
- ☐ Time limits and recorded agreements aid progress and accountability.
- ☐ Professionalism can, and should, involve service users and carers in active partnerships with practitioners.

KEY READING

Reid, W.J. (1992) *Task Strategies* New York: Columbia University Press

William Reid has been the leading task-centred practice researcher and developer. This book outlines the development and much of the detailed thinking behind task-centred practice, both in general terms and detailed enactment. While some of the ideas, especially around partnership models, have continued to develop, the book provides a solid foundation for studying task-centred practice.

CHAPTER 3

ANALYSE

OBJECTIVES

By the end of this chapter you should:

- Understand the central roles of partnership and communication in task-centred work
- Link the different stages of problem exploration to a metaphor of a newspaper page
- Recognise the important elements of goals within task-centred practice
- Follow the task implementation sequence
- Understand the value and roles of task review.

ANALYSING TASK-CENTRED PRACTICE

In Chapter 2 we introduced the work of two of the practitioners and the service users and carers whose endeavours will increasingly feature in *The Task-Centred Book*. This chapter adds more examples, takes key areas of task-centred practice and analyses the work in some detail.

Looking at examples like this provides a way to bring the real world of social work into the learning and teaching about task-centred practice. It also provides clearer material on exactly what is involved in carrying out some of the principles and practices of the model. We will be continuing to build on these and further practice examples as the book progresses.

The task-centred model, as we have seen, is founded on ideas of partnership, and ways in which the mandate for work and the goals of work can be clarified and agreed.

Communication is vital for this, and we begin the more detailed analysis of task-centred work by looking at partnership and communication, before moving on to problems, then to goals, then to tasks and review: a logical progression through the practice model.

TASK-CENTRED PRACTICE EXAMPLES

This chapter introduces three new task-centred examples. There is the work of Erica with Kelly (Portfolio B 2002), that of Margaret with Paula (Portfolio J 2002) and Gwen with John (Portfolio K 2002). These examples build on those introduced in Chapter 2; the new contexts introduced by the examples in this chapter are child abuse, disability and loss, and mental health. All the examples have elements of continuing care, none are 'simple' one-off pieces of work. The three practitioners also represent different stages of learning, with pre-qualified staff as well as qualified in this group, and with quite different lengths of experience.

Erica works in a Community Mental Health team and provided the following summary of the background of Kelly, who was referred to her from another service (Box 3.1).

BOX 3.1: KELLY, A SERVICE USER

Kelly was referred to the team by her psychiatrist. The reason for the referral was anxiety management and the psychiatrist was concerned that Kelly did not attend her outpatient appointments and was non-compliant with services . . . she was chronically agoraphobic and had rarely left the house for a three-year duration. She had not been out alone at all during this period.

Kelly has a history of childhood abuse – sexual, physical and emotional. In addition she suffers epilepsy and mild learning difficulties, meaning her literacy and numeracy were poor. Kelly is also hearing impaired having been born with only one ear drum, which is perforated.

As a result of her childhood experiences Kelly suffers nightmares and flashbacks and regularly dissociates. This impacts upon her ability to go out as she sees things flying at her and becomes paranoid that people are going to hurt her. In turn this leads to severe panic attacks, and many physical symptoms including fatigue, sickness and 'aching all over'.

She is looked after by Tina, providing virtually 24-hour care.

(Portfolio B 2002: 2.1)

Margaret works in an Adults Community team providing social services and she was approached directly by Paula for help (Box 3.2).

Gwen works in a Mental Health Support team as a pre-qualified assistant, and John was referred to her for support in the community following psychiatric hospital (Box 3.3).

BOX 3.2: PAULA, A SERVICE USER

Paula is a 29-year-old woman with cerebral palsy. For 28 years she has had all her physical needs met by her rather over-protective mother, with whom she has lived. When mum was diagnosed with terminal cancer in December, Paula approached the Community team for assistance with personal care and domestic tasks. I have been involved in the assessment and care management process with Paula since January. When mum entered the final stages of her illness, Paula asked for help with this transitional stage of her life. Mum died in late February and at Paula's request we began task-centred work in mid-March.

(Portfolio J 2002: 2.1)

BOX 3.3: JOHN, A SERVICE USER

A mental health referral was made from the ward in the psychiatric hospital regarding a patient who was ready for discharge but needed involvement from our agency prior to this.

John is a 54-year-old male who is diagnosed with schizophrenia. He had first been referred to our agency from the ward eight years ago as he was ready for discharge but had no accommodation to return to as a result of being evicted from his property. There were reports of unpaid bills and damage to property by the local housing department. Neighbours had reported incoherent ramblings of a religious nature which often needed police presence. There were incidents of self-harm and suicidal ideations.

(Portfolio K 2002: 2.1)

Under our headings of 'partnership and communication', 'problems', 'goals', and 'tasks and review', we shall follow the progress of these people through the task-centred model.

PARTNERSHIP AND COMMUNICATION

The basis of partnership, as we have noted in Chapter 2, is providing appropriate clarity about the mandate for intervention. This is not an easy task, often there is some blurring of exactly what is required and what is voluntary. Equally there may be some ambivalence about whether or not help is really being asked for, and how much it may be people's view that the problem is not with them but with someone else (who is not party to the discussion). But getting this right is vital, and getting it wrong will mean returning to it later. As Erica, in her analysis of what partnership and mandate meant in practice, noted:

> Prior to the training I did not spend as much time ensuring that the 'mandate' for the intervention was clear. I can now recognise that by spending more time at this stage fewer difficulties are likely to arise later on in the partnership

> when misunderstandings may occur. This means that future work should be more time effective and structured.
>
> (Portfolio B 2002: 2.5)

Working on this mandate issue, and establishing the basis for work will involve a careful balance from the practitioner in leading people to answer certain questions and being very careful to listen to their concerns and not guide them too much. There is a tightrope to be walked between what Reid has described as 'systematic' and 'responsive' communication (Reid and Epstein 1972: 127). The systematic communication aims to make progress through the model, guiding people to the next steps to be taken, and working logically through the different elements. Responsive communication expresses interest directly in people's comments, valuing them in their own right, not trying to shape but trying to build, not trying to move on, but showing empathy. Sometimes one mode will predominate, normally there will be some balance. It is not just the practitioner who will come to structure the work, as service users and carers become more aware of the stages in the model, and these should be outlined with as much clarity as possible, then they may well take the lead in structuring some discussions.

The feel of a partnership-based model, with a respect for the need for both responsive and systematic communication, should be something like that experienced by Erica in her work with Kelly and her carer, Tina:

> With my experience of task-centred working so far I have relished the opportunity to work in a structured manner with the reliance for progress lying equally between Kelly, Tina and myself. As I leave the session with an agreement to think about the problem to prioritise I am aware my service user and her carer will be doing the same as they have something positive to achieve from the process.
>
> (Portfolio B 2002: 2.5)

Communication to achieve this will involve a variety of techniques, drawing on skills that social work has valued and developed in many different settings. The way of talking needs to reflect partnership. It needs to be respectful, to value diversity, but it also needs to find ways to help people with the inevitable muddle that most social problems bring. People need to be helped to clarify their thoughts, and not to rush to answers, and often to move from problems being, as we have noted, 'all the fault of someone else'. Margaret expresses this well in her work with Paula:

> I am not always taking the time to ensure people understand the process and reasoning behind what I am doing . . . I have learned many very practical ideas that I can use in everyday work . . . asking people to reflect back to me what they understand that I have asked them . . . not offering solutions too soon as this avoids suggesting what people have already tried . . . shifting the focus of problems from the person to the interrelationship of behaviours.
>
> (Portfolio J 2002: 2.17)

Gwen, in her work with John, provides ideas about the ways that written communication, as well as verbal, can express the principles of partnership in a number of ways:

> We were both sat on the floor which worked well as it gave a feeling of equality. I made notes on A4 paper but shared these with John after each problem had been scanned. I asked John if he felt what I had written was a fair representation and if there was anything he wanted to add or alter.
>
> (Portfolio K 2002: 2.6)

Task-centred workers need to keep developing a good repertoire of skills of communication to achieve the partnership basis of the model (see Activity 3.1).

ACTIVITY 3.1: PRACTITIONER

Skill development

Think about the skills required in task-centred work. These could be ones which you think you already have, or they could be ones which you feel are not well developed at all. Make a list of those which you feel need developing. Ask a colleague who has done task-centred work if they will do the same, and compare lists. See what ways you could help each other to develop relevant skills, for example by shadowing, by shared reflection on work, by engaging supervisors.

Partnership is not about equality, it is about working towards common areas, and working in a joint and agreed manner. It involves 'putting cards on the table', as we have discussed about the mandate, and about seeking the best communication possible: communication that involves listening very carefully, but also guiding people through relevant model stages. The issue of power runs through partnership. Not in the patronising sense of empowering others, but in the sense of recognising who has what power, and whether it is appropriately discussed and used. In various ways practitioners and service users and carers will have power to:

- influence events
- obstruct events.

They will have power from:

- knowledge and information
- personal status
- social status (as a relatively powerful or powerless group)
- other sources (such as friends, family, or colleagues).

There is a complex power equation to be balanced, which will vary at different points in time, in task-centred work (see also Chapter 6). It is not necessarily a process of people gaining power by the end of the task-centred work, although the likelihood is that both parties will have done that, gaining, for example, skills and information from the work. John in his work with Gwen felt that the early stages changed his power, and that led to feelings of control quite early on.

> John expressed feelings of empowerment and gratitude for being able to select a problem important to him and to negotiate a goal from it. John said, 'I feel like I am gaining control of my situation before we have even started.'
>
> (Portfolio K 2002: 3.18)

Previous examples of 'partnership' working may have failed in the crucial elements of clarity which is needed, especially around goals, a point we will return to. Unless there are shared goals there will be no partnership. Erica found this a key part of her task-centred work:

> I find it refreshing to work in partnership with service users where the boundaries are so clear, and the goals the same for each of us.
>
> (Portfolio B 2002: 2.17)

We have been discussing partnership in situations where there is a reasonable degree of voluntarism about the work. But of course it is important to keep in mind the situations we covered in Chapter 2 of legal mandates for work, and that if people come to accept these as legitimate then task-centred work can begin, but if there is complete disagreement about this enforced work then models of work other than task-centred will be needed. If there can be no agreement about any element of the mandate then task-centred work cannot go ahead, and some form of supervision will be needed to enforce the legal mandate (see Activity 3.2).

ACTIVITY 3.2: MANAGER

Workload review: patterns of work

Do you have a clear idea of the workload levels for your staff? Is it possible for staff to undertake the 'short and fat' task-centred model of practice or do workload levels assume a 'long and thin' model? If more 'short and fat' work is to be done, will there be some recovery gaps between this more intensive work for staff to engage in learning or other activities?

There is an example answer in the Appendix.

Communication, so central to partnership, needs to be regular in task-centred work. Long gaps without communicating are likely to lead to drift away from the model, and not being able to respond to the events and circumstances that inevitably change as time goes by. Shorter gaps keep work more prominent, and are more likely to build motivation. Task-centred work is more likely to be 'short and fat' rather than 'long and thin' in its structure.

Meetings between Paula and Margaret reflected this: 'I feel that meeting weekly has kept a momentum and motivation going for both the service users and myself' (Portfolio J 2002: 5.41).

However, as we discussed earlier, it is not just regular conversations that are a key part of the work, so is regular written material, or some other regular form of record. Recording reminds people, it informs people, it clarifies what is meant, and helps to generate accountability. Reminding, informing, clarifying and providing accounts are all important elements of task-centred work (see Activity 3.3).

Margaret felt that the need to think about

> participation, clarity and focus ... compelled me to think again about ways I can write my regular recording in partnership with service users ...

> I have increasingly used summaries in my regular practice and given the service user a copy.
>
> (Portfolio J 2002: 5.44)

ACTIVITY 3.3: SUPERVISOR

Developing records

- What records do you see in supervision?
- How might these best support the task-centred model?
- How can you help staff to engage in joint recording with service users and carers?
- Are there innovative ideas about recording that you could make a note of and share across your supervision sessions?

PROBLEMS

An urgent and pressing problem at the point of first contact between practitioner and service user and carer may need to be dealt with before work on the mandate and on problem exploration begins. The need to assure safety, or deal with an urgent issue of care should take priority. There is a sense in which, in the technical terminology of task-centred work, this will be a 'pre-problem' piece of work. Helping, but not helping in an organised way as part of the model. Handling the housing eviction, or the need for linking promptly with a health worker, is of course the sensible thing to do if it is urgently needed. After this the task-centred work can begin.

In task-centred work, if the mandate is a voluntary one, people decide the priority within the problems scanned. Practitioners should provide good advice to help people decide but ultimately the decision lies with the service user and carer. Gwen spent some time working on this issue of priority with John. Here is her analysis of this work:

> We finally, after much discussion, agreed upon a selected problem to work on. John felt that he would like to go out and experience more activities . . . I personally felt that this might not be the most appropriate problem to work on. I got the impression from what John continually said that his appearance was the main issue . . . when I raised this with John, as delicately as I could, John looked and sounded quite offended . . . John explained to me that he could not choose this as the problem to work on as he felt his appearance could not be changed. When I tried to take this further John refused, saying, 'There is nothing I can do about it'. John and I agreed to put this discussion behind us and focus on the selected problem.
>
> (Portfolio K 2002: 2.10)

Of course, if there had also been a legally mandated problem, that would have been added to the work, and as we shall note again when we come to discuss goals, if this legally mandated problem could not be accepted at all, then a model of supervision rather than of task-centred work would need to be followed.

Problems may also be added because the practitioner needs to suggest them, based on their professional knowledge and expertise. Suggesting problems to add is a delicate task, and to suggest without enforcing is a skill in itself. Here is Erica, suggesting a problem to be added to Kelly's work, and carefully discussing the reasons for the suggested addition:

> At the end of Kelly and Tina's descriptions of the difficulties faced I added an additional problem I felt they encountered. This was readily accepted by the participants. I discussed my view that Kelly was suffering from poor motivation in certain areas of life and that this could be impacting upon some of the problems scanned this session. Once I explained symptoms and possible causes of poor motivation they agreed that this was indeed something that required considering along with other scanned problems and it was added to the list.
>
> (Portfolio B 2002: 2.11)

Erica gives Kelly and Tina the chance to reject the idea, but they are prepared to go along with it. Task-centred work is a constant process of judging how much to press a point, how far to go with a suggestion, and how far to be responsive and reflective.

Producing a priority problem, or problems, involves the stages outlined in Chapter 2: a scan of all relevant problems, additions of problems practitioners see or that are legally mandated, some details, a summary in people's own words, and then the priority order.

The end product of this process will produce problems of different priority, and will give quotes and a story to each. This is similar to the front page of a newspaper, with its main headlines, and its lower level stories, and with its quotes and its more detailed coverage. This metaphor of the newspaper front page is useful to help people to understand this process, and it may be that presenting the result of the problem scan and exploration in this way will work well (see Activity 3.4). Experience shows that people find this a very satisfactory and understandable way to present the results of the problem work. Of course if there are literacy problems the 'newspaper' page could be read out, or greatly simplified to bullet points.

Perhaps the key element to emphasise is the use of the actual words of service users and carers in the construction of this page: real quotes from real life showing the essence of what is meant without professional jargon. Helping to shape these is a skill that involves the minimum of shaping and the maximum of helping simply to clarify meaning. Ultimately these are people's own words. Here are some examples:

- 'I can't get better because I can't get to see the doctor or psychiatrist.'
- 'If I do go to sleep I wake up a lot in the night. Sometimes I can't even get to sleep in the first place.'
- 'Kelly relies heavily on me and sometimes I think she is more capable than she acts. She does not react when she sees how hard I am finding it to cope, Tina says.'

(Portfolio B 2002: 2.8)

ACTIVITY 3.4: LEARNER

Reviewing your work: the newspaper metaphor

- Use the newspaper metaphor discussed above with three of your current pieces of work.
- Does your work readily adapt to the 'newspaper' approach? What aspects were relatively easy and which more difficult? Why?
- What changes would you need to make to make best use of this approach?

GOALS

The problems to be worked on ('things that are wrong'), assuming there is a mandate to do this, will lead a task-centred worker to jointly develop with service users and carers a goal or goals ('things that are wanted'). There is a limit to the number of problems that should be given a priority to develop into goals, too many means a lack of proper examination of priorities and a lack of focus to the work, but more than one may often be needed. A maximum of two, or perhaps three, is probably a good rule, for the problems to be worked on, and if there is more than one then the overall number of goals being aimed at should probably not exceed three either. Different situations will call for different combinations for problems and goals, for example one priority problem with up to three goals, two priority problems with two goals for one and one for another, or perhaps three problems and one goal each.

Of course there will be an opportunity to re-contract at a later stage with a new agreement and new goals if needed, although this should not be done lightly.

Problem exploration can involve covering a wide variety of problems, and this needs handling with great sensitivity. Generating priority problems will help to avoid problem exploration feeling overwhelming. Making clear links to goals also will help. Moving more quickly onto goals may be needed, and moving carefully back and forth between problems and goals may be part of the necessary sensitivity to avoiding the feeling of there being 'too many' problems.

Erica recognised and analysed the issue of needing to avoid the negative side of careful problem exploration in her work with Kelly and Tina:

> I believe that the problem exploration was far less complicated in this instance than I anticipated, largely due to Tina's presence and reassurance throughout the process. However, the session still caused Kelly distress and she had a feeling of despondency and loss of worth at the amount of problems she faced.
>
> In hindsight I would have perhaps helped the process be a more positive experience had I spent longer discussing the outcomes of the work at the beginning of the session.
>
> (Portfolio B 2002: 2.12)

Goals ideally need to be as SMART as possible, as discussed in Chapter 2. But getting this degree of clarity is difficult, and again a careful judgement needs to be made not to overwhelm the process by labouring too long to avoid fuzzy goals. Using the words of service users and carers may sometimes conflict with the need to avoid fuzziness as well. On the other hand clear goals are important to make the work successful. This is another delicate tightrope to walk for the task-centred practitioner, and it was experienced acutely by Margaret in her work with Paula:

> Paula selected two very different problems and identified goals. The first problem was her frustration at her lack of independence. Paula herself stated her goal as wanting to rebuild her life and work towards a future. I certainly felt this goal was feasible, desirable and linked with her problem. I felt the goal was 'fuzzy' and needed more definition. On analysis, I feel I did not want to move away from Paula's stated goal because I felt keeping her own words linked with her motivation . . . however, I did feel that I needed to get Paula to be more specific so that we had something against which to measure progress. I introduced the idea of a success indicator . . . Paula then stated more clear statements, such as 'the house will be in my name' which we will be able to look back at in six weeks time to establish whether the goals have been achieved.
>
> (Portfolio J 2002: 3.23)

Goals should ideally have strong elements of the following:

- *motivation*: to achieve them
- *feasibility*: practical, can be done, do not involve too much commitment of others
- *desirability*: ethical, reasonable, decent
- *alleviation*: genuinely contributing in the eyes of the service user and carer to problem reduction.

Goals that are SMART, and that are positive in these four areas will be the best foundation for task-centred work.

TASKS AND REVIEW

Tasks are the key activities to make progress towards the goals. They need to be done by the practitioner and by service users and carers, and they need to be reviewed. It is this process of action and review that helps to show progress and to indicate what skills or resources might be needed.

Once problems, goals and time limits are established then some initial tasks will be generated. These will form the first of the steps towards the goal(s). At the next session they will be reviewed.

Once the task phase of work begins, each session follows a sequence:

- a quick review of the problem(s)
- a review of the tasks that have been agreed: have they been done and with what results?
- an assessment of progress towards the goal(s)
- the generation of new tasks.

Please turn to Chapter 7 for more detailed consideration of this process.

Erica, working with Kelly, found that the work on tasks was cumulatively positive:

> The review stage enabled me to concentrate on each step she made to reach her goal and to praise her accordingly. In Kelly's past she has not received much positive feedback, and so this was an important and rewarding process. Kelly's confidence began to increase and her self-image to improve. She began to believe in her abilities and this enabled her to feel more positive about the next set of tasks she planned to undertake.
>
> (Portfolio B 2002: 4.44)

Because tasks are smaller steps towards the goal they may be very effective in helping people tackle things they have been avoiding, and John clearly thought this:

> John found it easier to complete a task at a time and felt highly motivated after each task was completed. John stated, 'I have wanted to do this for such a long time but kept putting it off because it felt like such a big thing.'
>
> (Portfolio K 2002: 5.30)

To be successful, tasks, like other elements of the model, need to be clearly understood by both the practitioner and service user and carer. The practice that is the task needs to be clear (*what*), the reason for the task (contribution to movement towards the goal) needs to be evident (*why*), and the person doing the task needs to have the capacity to do it (*how*).

Ideally tasks need to be undertaken by both practitioners and service users and carers, perhaps with some overall balance, but certainly with an eye to helping to develop people's skills. Suggestions for tasks are usually more from the practitioner than from the service user and carer, although this may change as work progresses. There is, as usual in task-centred work, a delicate balance between suggesting and influencing. Workers should be suggesting tasks, and exploring their relevance and likely contribution to progress, they should not be stipulating them or unduly pushing people into doing them.

Tasks need to be agreed, then they need to be carried out. It is possible to have in-session tasks (making a phone call to find information or move a decision on, would be a common example), but perhaps more commonly tasks are undertaken between sessions. Tasks, as we have noted in Chapter 2, can be one-off, individual, shared, recurring or reciprocal. Whatever the version, the task is more likely to be successful if the practitioner follows through the Task Planning and Implementation Sequence. This was developed and tested in the early 1970s as part of the research to provide the foundations of the model (Reid 1975) and has been further developed since then (Reid 2000). Please turn to Chapter 6 (page 122) for more details and see also Box 4.7.

The Task Planning and Implementation Sequence provides the following steps:

- choosing the task (different options generated)
- agreeing the task
- planning details
- enhancing commitment
- considering possible obstacles
- providing guidance (coaching, modelling, etc.) where appropriate and summarising.

There was, for example, some need for confidence building with Kelly to enhance her commitment to the tasks:

> Kelly had little faith in her ability to succeed and was so terrified of failing that she began to be anxious and the process started to have a negative effect on her mental health. Hence it was necessary to undertake confidence building alongside the process to enable it to succeed.
>
> (Portfolio B 2002: 4.32)

With Paula the enhancement of commitment was briefer, but session tasks showed obstacles which would need to be taken into account, and overcome, if tasks between sessions were to be successful:

> Paula found the telephone number for the wheelchair company and called them while I was present. This revealed that the company no longer services Paula's model of wheelchair. This then meant that we needed to go to the phonebook and look for service engineers . . . we identified that Paula cannot physically hold the phonebook and write numbers from it, so I read out some numbers and Paula wrote them down.
>
> (Portfolio J 2002: 4.29)

Once commitment is firm, and plans are made, and obstacles analysed it may be necessary to help with the preparation for task work by undertaking modelling and/or rehearsal and/or guided practice. These three activities are very useful but often practitioners seem to skip over them. Maybe they are not a regular part of the non-task-centred repertoire, and maybe practitioners even find the idea of showing or guiding people in tasks a bit embarrassing; so practitioners leave them out despite the great value placed on them by service users and carers. These are very important activities and should not be missed out if they are likely to be at all relevant.

Modelling will involve showing directly how to do something, rehearsal, as the name suggests, involves trying out a task away from the real situation, and guided practice involves the practitioner working alongside people as they undertake the task or part-task.

Here is Erica, helping in this phase of task work, with some modelling and some guided practice:

> By undertaking the task myself while Kelly and Tina observed we were able to ascertain that we all had the same understanding and expectation of the task, which also enhanced the summarising. In addition by undertaking the task with Kelly and Tina I was able to observe areas of potential difficulty and then work through them prior to Kelly and Tina doing the task alone. Hence we looked at positive coping strategies such as controlled breathing to increase the potential of the task being completed successfully.
>
> (Portfolio B 2002: 4.37)

At the end of these elements the practitioner needs to summarise the tasks that have been agreed, and any ideas for helping to make sure they are successful (see Activity 3.5).

ACTIVITY 3.5: TRAINER

Encouraging specific skills: modelling, guided practice and rehearsal

Experience shows that the use of modelling, guided practice and rehearsal is low despite the value of these activities. Devise a brief training programme that will help practitioners to make better use of these three processes.

Carrying out the task work will help to show areas of strengths, and should aid in developing strengths. It may also indicate problems that need to be overcome, skills that need to be learnt. Each task needs to be reviewed properly. A score for the task, applied of course equally to practitioner tasks as to service user and carer ones, is helpful. 'Four out of five' is clearly good progress, and shows the good progress in a way that is very clear. Conversely 'two out of five' shows difficulties. A score of 'nought' for not undertaken, also makes the lack of work notably evident. As we have repeated so often these scores should be done in a positive and respectful manner, with sensitivity and care. They are not a test score, they do show a number of things that are vital indicators for task-centred work. They also hold practitioners to account in a way they often, initially, find uncomfortable, but accountability is important to partnership.

If tasks are undone, or partially done, what does this indicate? It could indicate simply problems of time and access. It could indicate more obstacles than anticipated, and these need working on. It could indicate the wrong task, and this should always be considered. If tasks are regularly undone it may indicate that the goal is not really one that is wanted, and this could trigger a more comprehensive review of the work than normal (see Activity 3.6).

ACTIVITY 3.6: SERVICE USER AND CARER

Giving feedback

- Box 3.4 has a set of questions which have been developed to help people to analyse their experience of task-centred practice and to give feedback about how they found it.
- Are there any other questions which you would like to be asked that you would add to this list?
- Would you suggest changes to some of the questions that are already there and, if so, what would these be?

In Chapter 7 (Boxes 7.6 and 7.7) you can see examples of two sets of questions and the answers which a service user gave.

At the end of the agreed period of work there needs to be a final review of progress. It is unusual for work to completely meet the exact goal or goals agreed. However, the progress often means a great deal even if it does not go as far as was once hoped. The work should have resulted in enhanced skills and knowledge, and probably new skills and knowledge for the service users and carers, and perhaps the putting in place of support services of various kinds. The ideal is perhaps for the practitioner to 'do themselves out of a job'.

This end point is a time to consider possible extension. More of the same is unlikely to be ideal except in unusual circumstances where things have gone wrong because of outside events. In these circumstances though it is probably best to renegotiate, perhaps quite briefly, maybe take a break, and start again. However, a new agreement is quite possible if there is new work to be done.

BOX 3.4: SERVICE USER'S EVALUATION

These questions are asked because I would like you to let me know what you think about the work we have done together, and to help me to improve my work. This will help us both to get the best out of the ending of our work.

- *The beginning*
  Looking back to the beginning of our work, why do you think I got involved with you?
- *Our written agreement*
  What did you think about our written agreement? Did you like this style of work? For example, did it help to use pens and paper in our work together?
- *The goal*
  How near to your goal are you? What tells you how near you are to your goal? How near to your goal do other people think you are?
- *In general*
  Looking over the work we have done together, what was most useful? What was least useful – could we have done some things differently?
- *The future*
  Now that we have finished our work together, will you try this way of doing things without me?

The final review is an important stage, it should not be rushed, and it should be treated very seriously as an assessment by all parties of how things have gone, including whether or not, with hindsight, this really was the right problem to work on. It is important, as well, to review the progress toward the goal, whether or not others might think there has been progress towards the goal, views about this way of working, and future needs.

Overall people are very positive about task-centred practice. Here are some comments from the people we have been hearing from in this chapter:

> John felt that the model had helped him a lot. He felt the tasks and incremental steps had helped him build up the confidence to go for a coffee alone. John said he felt involved all the way through the process and felt listened to.
>
> (Portfolio K 2002: 5.29)

> Kelly thinks that the work was 'great'. She said she appreciated the structure and support it offered and felt she concentrated more on positives and success than failures and negatives. Tina agreed with this.
>
> (Portfolio B 2002: 4.48)

> Undoubtedly I feel there have been benefits secondary to the work on the goal itself. Kelly's achievements appear to have transcended into every area of her life and has certainly had a positive effect on many of her scanned problems . . . sleeping has improved although still suffers nightmares . . . more motivated throughout the day . . . making a certain amount of cups of tea for her and for Tina . . . generally happier with herself.
>
> (Portfolio B 2002: 5.51)

> In reviewing tasks with Paula I have learned how very determined and committed she is to her goals, she has completed each task except those where she has been reliant on assistance from other agencies. This has indicated to me that perhaps other people do not take her seriously enough to act on promises they make her . . . I need to take this on board in my dealings with other agencies, and take every opportunity to challenge poor service given to all people with disabilities.
>
> (Portfolio J 2002: 4.34)

All parties to task-centred work are likely to change and learn through their experience of working on the mandate, problems, goals, time limits, tasks and reviews. They will need to analyse their situation carefully, they will need to analyse what matters and what does not, and what works and what does not. The analysis of the practitioners and the service users and carers presented in this chapter provides the foundation for task-centred practice. Chapters 4 and 5 will move from this foundation to the business of teaching and learning professional practice, before Chapter 6 again brings us back to the detail of task-centred practice.

KEY POINTS

- ☐ Task-centred practice involves the movement from problem to goal.
- ☐ Using service users' and carers' own words to describe problems and goals is a vital aid to partnership and to clarity of purpose.
- ☐ The mandate for practice must be as clear as possible to all concerned.
- ☐ Goals need to be as SMART as possible, and ideally to have strong elements of motivation, feasibility, desirability and problem alleviation.
- ☐ Tasks are most likely to be effective if a set of actions, called the task implementation sequence, is followed.
- ☐ The final review of the work is an important stage, providing an accountable end and also a developmental process in its own right.

KEY READING

Reid, W. J. (1975) A test of a task-centred approach *Social Work* **20** (January): 3–9

The development and origin of the task implementation sequence can be found in this article, which provides a lucid summary of the logic behind the development of different parts of task-centred practice, and also further details of the sequence.

Tolson, E., Reid, W. J. and Garvin, C. (1994) *Generalist Practice: A Task-Centered Approach* New York: Columbia University Press

A good outline of the task-centred model, which then takes it clearly beyond work with individuals into families, groups and communities, is provided in this substantial textbook.

CHAPTER 4

TEACH

OBJECTIVES

By the end of this chapter you should:

- Understand how to teach task-centered practice effectively
- Know how to use a range of materials to teach task-centered practice
- Know the best structure and shape for teaching task-centered practice
- Teach people to identify strengths
- Differentiate between problems, goals and tasks.

TEACHING TASK-CENTRED PRACTICE

The task-centred method became known in the UK after the publication of *Task-Centred Casework* (Reid and Epstein 1972) in the United States, and was soon incorporated into social work qualifying programmes. However, it was the National Institute of Social Work (NISW) which developed a specific training model in task-centred practice to take to social work agencies and probation services across the UK in the late 1970s and early 1980s (Atherton 1982; McCaughan and Vickery 1982). At the same time, Jane Gibbons, Matilda Goldberg and their colleagues were conducting action research projects in which participants were taught the task-centred method, with evaluation of their subsequent practice (Gibbons *et al.* 1979; Goldberg *et al.* 1984a).

We developed the training model further, with the experience of several programmes in social work and probation agencies in England, Scotland and Wales during the 1980s. Since the mid–1990s, the programme has been established as an option for continuing professional development at pre- and post-qualifying levels. The task-centred training programme has been accredited with post-qualifying credits, with an assessment element provided by a portfolio (Doel *et al.* 2002). Much of *The Task-Centred Book* is informed by the experience of these training programmes, from which the materials in the boxes in this chapter are derived, as well as the quotes from task-centred practitioners.

A STRUCTURE TO TEACH TASK-CENTRED PRACTICE

Teaching a method of professional practice requires tutors to consider a number of complex issues. It is not just a question of how learners can best understand the 'blue-print' of the method, but of developing their ability to put this knowledge into practice. This teaching and learning does not take place in a vacuum, but is highly influenced by the availability of time and space, support from colleagues and line managers, the emotional dimension of the learning (Atkins 2002), and the relevance to the learner's everyday experiences in practice. It must challenge existing practice to induce change, but not so radically that it is rejected.

Box 4.1 illustrates a structure which, after several refinements, we have found helpful in promoting successful learning and application to practice. It incorporates a number of principles which we will consider below.

Preparation

Participants must be aware of the expectations and demands that the training course will make on them. Although the model is deceptively simple on paper, much energy is needed to follow the task-centred method systematically; this message is reinforced all the more convincingly by participants of previous programmes, who take part in the information session held about two months before the programme begins. This gives potential applicants the opportunity to find out more about the programme before committing themselves on the basis of an informed choice.

Support

It is difficult to sustain the encouragement and enthusiasm beyond the workshop and into the workplace; even the following day those positive workshop experiences can seem a distant memory as the phones ring and other demands take precedence. Having a partner in training who has shared these experiences and who returns with you to the workplace is likely to reinforce commitment. Sticking 'what we are going to do' flipchart sheets side by side on the office wall takes the workshop learning directly into the workplace and shows mutual solidarity. Presentations to colleagues can widen this support and, indeed, is essential where there is shared care for people:

> [There] were problems that related to support staff [working with the service user] understanding the concept of task-centred practice and then employing it into [their] working practices.
>
> (Portfolio I 2003: 2.2)

BOX 4.1: A STRUCTURED, HALF-YEAR PROGRAMME

- *Intro* **Information session** *(two months prior to programme start, e.g. July)*
  For interested practitioners and their supervisors to meet the tutors and some past participants in the training programme; presentation of the programme and opportunity for questions, etc.; examples of successful task-centred portfolios; how to apply to the training programme.
- *Part 1* **Week 1** *(e.g. late September)*
  First *consultation*: one hour each for (paired) practitioners and their supervisors (line managers).
  Initial reading, preparation and discussion of mutual expectations.
- *Part 2* **Week 3** *(e.g. early October)*
  First *workshop* for all the supervisors (half-day).
  The theoretical framework and value base of task-centred practice; principles and model: agreement, mandate, tasks and review; supervision and practice development in task-centred practice.
- First *workshop* for all the practitioners (two days)
  The theoretical framework and value base of task-centred practice (TCP); misconceptions about TCP; its scope and limitations; the five phases: mandate, exploring problems, negotiating a written agreement, task work, and review; evaluating and ending work: task-centred work in context (putting the method to work in a particular work setting with a particular user group); gathering evidence for the task-centred portfolio.
- *Part 3* **Week 6** *(e.g. late October)*
  Second *consultation*: one hour each for (paired) practitioners and their supervisors (line managers).
  Consider progress with the task-centred work *(By this stage we hope you will have completed the problem exploration stage and come to a written agreement with the service user(s) in at least one case)*; practitioners present a draft of the first Unit of their portfolio.
- *Part 4* **Week 8** *(e.g. mid-November)*
  Second *workshop* for all the practitioners (one day).
  Progress report on using the model in practice; sharing successes and rehearsing difficulties.
- *Part 5* **Week 11** *(e.g. early December)*
  Joint *workshop* for everyone (half-day).
  Consolidation of the use of the model in practice and supervision; presentations.
- *Part 6* **Week 16** *(e.g. mid-January)*
  Final review workshop for everyone (half-day).
  To review progress on task-centred practice and supervision; to review the model and the training programme; plans to help sustain task-centred work; guidance on the submission of the portfolio.
- **Week 26** *(e.g. end of March)*
  Final submission of portfolio.

It is important to have the support of the supervisor or line manager. The one-to-one consultations in the training programme are, in effect, 'two-to-three' between the two course tutors and the two paired practitioners and their supervisor ('two-to-four' if each practitioner has a different supervisor). This way, line managers hear directly about the time and energy necessary for success and are involved in considering how this can be made available. This should help prevent the hostility which some practitioners have reported experiencing on return from training courses (Rushton and Martyn 1990). The managers are implicated in discussions about the benefits which the course will bring, and they take part in a crash course to become more familiar with what their supervisees will be doing.

Timing

The programme can never be quite the right length or come at quite the right pace for every participant, but the outline structure (Box 4.1) has been refined over many trials to provide the best common denominator. There needs to be sufficient time between the initial application and the first consultation for pairings to be negotiated and preparatory reading to be completed. With good notice, participants can keep the dates free in their diaries so that they do not miss any components.

The 'sandwiches' of consultations and workshops are timed so that participants will have useful material to bring to both; after the first consultation they are advised to start an immediate search for likely referrals of service users so they will be in a position to start the task-centred work immediately after the first workshop. If the momentum is lost it takes much more effort to retrieve it. The relationship of workshop to consultation allows these kind of linkages to be made:

> After discussing the selected problem [in consultation with the task-centred tutors], it was felt that the selected problem in some respects was a little too fuzzy and needed to be clearer in order for the goal to be determined and measurable. When I took this back to the service user at the next session, he agreed and between us we discussed what he would like to achieve. He spoke of how in the past he used to go for a coffee in a café in the centre of [Townville] and would like to be able to do so again.
>
> (Portfolio K 2002: 2.3)

At the other end of the programme, it is not easy to judge how much time each participant will need to complete their portfolio of evidence. Events may have conspired to prevent the completion of a case (preferably two), with people's circumstances changing, and a need to start afresh late in the programme. Nevertheless, even when a case has faltered half-way through, there is usually much learning which can be transferred to a start with new people.

Assessment

More evidence is needed, but it seems that the participants' work on their portfolios reinforces the teaching and consolidates their learning. The portfolio template follows a parallel route to the work itself, and is 'signposted' (Doel *et al.* 2002) by a series of questions which indicate descriptive responses, then analytical and finally reflective responses. We refer to some of these portfolios regularly in this book, since the work they document is highly illustrative of the task-centred method in practice.

Continuing professional development is becoming a matter of professional obligation rather than personal choice, and it will be interesting to see if learners' enthusiasm is affected when assessment is seen as a necessary chore for credits. This has not yet been observed.

CLASS-BASED MODELS OF TEACHING TASK-CENTRED PRACTICE

The material in the boxes and the activities in this chapter are relevant to teaching task-centred practice in the classroom as well as agency-based training. However, the structure of class-based teaching needs to reflect the fact that students will not have the opportunity to practice the method, unless they are concurrently on placement. They may need more opportunities for role play to rehearse the different stages of the model, and it is useful to invite experienced task-centred practitioners to lead small groups, so that useful links can be made with practice. Qualifying social work courses in the UK are, rightly or wrongly, 'eclectic', so task-centred practice is often just one of many methods appearing briefly in 'social work methods' modules. The growing focus on evidence-based practice suggests that there needs to be greater discrimination between methods and approaches, with emphasis on those practice methods which are found to be most effective and empowering. We believe that task-centred practice is more than just *primus inter pares*.

The key to a successful transition from understanding in the class to application in the field is the strength of the links with practice teachers (student supervisors) who have knowledge and experience of using the model systematically. This is why continuing professional development in agencies is crucial to the cycle; at present, 'we used a task-centred approach' is a far more common sighting in the student's portfolio of placement work than it is in the reality of practice. The links would also be reinforced if task-centred supervision becomes a favoured method of practice teaching (Caspi and Reid 2002), to help make 'practice teachers . . . more confident and competent at articulating their practice assumptions' (Brodie 1993: 85).

FIRST STEPS

A baseline of the learner's knowledge is a useful starting point. Complete Activity 4.1 now and return to it when you have completed your first piece of task-centred practice. In what ways has your definition changed, if at all?

ACTIVITY 4.1: ALL

Defining task-centered practice: a starting point

In one or two sentences, how would you define task-centred practice?

Another first step is to consider what a 'practice method' is. It is our experience that students and practitioners are often intimidated or confused by the relationship of theories to models to methods to techniques (Stepney and Ford 2000: viii). Box 4.2 can form the basis of a handout to introduce learners to the notion of *practice method*, in relation to all forms of practice, not just task-centred practice. However, if we accept that these are necessary components of a practice method, it becomes apparent that there are perhaps not many methods in reality. For example, though we can speak of a psychosocial approach, is there a psychosocial method as such?

BOX 4.2: WHAT IS A PRACTICE METHOD?

Five components of a practice method

- A practice method is a way of working which is *systematic*.
- It is based on a particular body of knowledge, perhaps organised into *a theory*.
- The method should have been *tested* in practice and *researched*, so that it can be refined and modified.
- A method should be explicit about its *value base*.
- It should have a *practice technology*, which lets us know how to use it in practice. There might be a number of associated *techniques, such as paradoxical injunction* in some methods of family counselling, and the Task Planning and Implementation Sequence (TPIS) in task-centred practice.

A method is not something which we can choose to use; whenever we work with people using social work services we are using some kind of 'method'. What differs is the extent to which the method is systematic or not, explicit or implicit, tested or untested, etc. We have a responsibility to make our methods as open as possible to people we use them with.

It is important early on for teachers and learners to discover how the learner's current practice fits with and differs from the task-centred approach. This covers practical issues such as the shape of encounters with people, which we have characterised as 'short and fat' or 'long and thin' (Doel and Marsh 1992: 90).

The short, fat encounters are more conducive to task-centred work. In addition to the practicalities of time to implement and reflect on task-centred practice, there is the question of the learner's current value base. If we rely on declared values we will learn little: how many practitioners declare that their practice is discriminatory, oppressive and not based on partnership? It is necessary to help learners to articulate the assumptions, working hypotheses and practice prescriptions which guide their work (Wedenoja *et al.* 1988). This is not an inquisitorial attempt to prove that they *are* discriminatory and oppressive, but to understand that to develop what is truly 'a partnership' is an ideal and that actual practice is steeped in dilemma and compromise. The worker's unspoken guiding principles have a huge impact on practice, and these may or may not support task-centred values of partnership.

This mix of assumption, tacit theory and working hypothesis can be made manifest by drawing on a concrete example, such as Activity 4.2.

ACTIVITY 4.2: PRACTITIONER

Working hypotheses: 'The Dales'

Janet Dale is a married woman, aged 23. Her husband, John, is about the same age. They have two children, Katie aged 4 and Jamie aged 2, and they live in John's parents' council house. Although the furniture is shabby, the house is clean and relatively tidy.

Janet has spent much of the last four years in and out of the psychiatric hospital, spending one period in the secure ward. Recently, she has been attending the day hospital from the psychiatric hospital. She has now run home from the day hospital. Her mother-in-law, Jean, took her back to the hospital, but she has run home again. She is now quite calm. The family want her to stay home and hope she won't have to return to hospital.

Janet and John are a quiet, unassuming couple. Her father-in-law, Graham Dale, has the same qualities. Her mother-in-law is a very capable, effective person who has run the house and looked after the children and the two men completely in recent years, despite advancing arthritis. Janet has been home from time to time and, according to Jean, has been unable to do anything for herself. She is frightened of going to the shops and, despite Jean's attempts to show her what to do, is unable to do everyday domestic chores.

- What two questions do you want to ask? And of whom?

Later:

- What hypotheses have you made to explain what is happening here?

Having taught task-centred practice with several hundred practitioners and students, it is our experience that people have very different, yet strongly held notions of causality which they use, often at a subliminal level, to explain what they see. Moreover, many people seem to need little information (no more than given in Activity 4.2) before drawing heavily on these explanations. Professing a strong commitment to the value of a 'strengths' model frequently does not inhibit working hypotheses which are actually quite the opposite. The following views tend to predominate:

- 'Jean is a controlling woman, manipulating the rest of the family.'
- 'John has opted out of family life and shows no interest in the care of his children.'
- 'Janet is a victim.'

However, the following working hypotheses are seldom voiced:

- 'Jean stepped into the breach to keep the family together, despite her increasing disability.'
- 'John has stood by his wife and managed to hold a job together even in the face of all the stresses of the last few years.'
- 'Janet has taken her destiny into her own hands.'

These are all facets of the same reality, but practitioners need to learn how to integrate them into a wider understanding. Since many service users and carers are also often ill-equipped at identifying the strengths, practitioners need to be skilled at reframing to illuminate these strengths. Language is all-important in this process: put at its simplest, it is the difference between 'Janet ran away from hospital' and 'Janet ran back to home' (which was a notable feat for someone with agoraphobic tendencies).

An exercise such as 'The Dales' exposes the links between practical social work and philosophical approaches to notions of causality, evidence and meaning. Indeed, teleological thinking is in evidence throughout the portfolios of task-centred practice, including this following example about the 'causes' of task-centred practice itself!

> The task-centred model has developed over the past two decades because of the lack of methods of practice originating within social work produced by social workers and social work researchers.
>
> (Portfolio K 2002: 1.1)

The two statements below are presented as facts, though they are statements of opinion:

> If she felt more in control she would feel less depressed.
>
> (Portfolio G 2000: 2.3)

> Due to his lack of insight, John did not see the point of having an injection when he was not ill.
>
> (Portfolio K 2002: 2.2)

'The Dales' exercise helps practitioners to see these kinds of statements as working hypotheses and to consider how the strengths dimension can be included. The task-centred system of careful recording of the person's view of the world does ensure that, even among the litter of working hypotheses, there is the glint of the users' and carers' own meanings:

> Due to his lack of insight, John did not see the point of having an injection when he was not ill. *John stated he also lacked the confidence to go for, and the funds to pay for, the prescription.*
>
> (Portfolio K 2002: 2.2 – our italics)

Relating to life experience

Quite early on in the teaching programme, learners start to make associations between the task-centred model as a professional model of practice, and the problem-solving methods which they use in their own lives.

> I want to train to be a social worker (goal). I intend to do this by the time I am 30 years old (time limit) and I intend to gain more work experience while completing courses such as Task-Centred Practice (tasks), which will give me more credit towards achieving my goal.
>
> (Portfolio K 2002: 3.1)

> Looking back over the last six years I have built my own career using a task-centred approach. I had a problem – dissatisfied with working as an unqualified residential social worker – the goal was to be a qualified social worker

> in a children and families community team. I gave myself four years to achieve this.
>
> (Portfolio D 2002: 3.1)

These associations reinforce the notion that service users and carers are fellow citizens whose lives have brought them into contact with social services. Social work differs from many professions in that, virtually by definition, almost all the people who use its services, voluntarily or not, experience some degree of relative poverty, discrimination and disadvantage. The task-centred method helps remind practitioners of the strengths which have enabled people to endure these experiences, to really listen to their stories, and to work with people's innate problem-solving capacities.

AN EXAMPLE TRAINING COURSE

In Box 4.1 we presented a suggested structure for a programme to teach task-centred practice. In the next pages we consider the content of such a programme in more detail, with Boxes 4.3 to 4.10 providing materials which can be used to support the learning.

Exploring problems

Having taught about the general notion of a practice method (Box 4.2) and related task-centred practice to the learner's existing knowledge, values and experience, it is time to teach the details of the model. As we outlined in Chapter 2, the first stage beyond introduction and the mandate for the work is one of exploring problems. Most learners will be familiar with the general process of exploring problems, since it is closely related to many of the activities often referred to as 'assessment'. However, this closeness has many disadvantages. Like English-speakers from Britain and North America, their supposedly common language is the more dangerous precisely because they are not aware of the differences.

One of the greatest difficulties in learning to explore problems is so simple that it is hard to credit: the ability just to listen to what the person has to say about their problems. Of course, the listening needs to be focused and directed. In other words, it is punctuated with questions, etc. by the practitioner to help guide the person through the five stages (Box 4.3). However, experienced practitioners in particular can find it difficult not to work with a hidden agenda of the problems which they or others have identified, or with the agency's assessment schedule at the front of their mind (and, therefore, in their ears).

Practising the exploring problems stage by using rehearsal, first in a large group (with the tutor modelling as practitioner), then in small groups of three, is an effective way of easing the necessary shift. It is more effective to use a case example in which no one is involved ('The Dales' can be used, for example), since this avoids defensive justification of actions already taken and helps learners to step outside the well-worn track. Having each trio seated around a piece of flipchart paper tracking each stage of the problem exploration, is an effective way of helping learners to understand how this differs from their usual practices. Each person in the trio should have the opportunity to rehearse the practitioner, play the user or carer and be the observer. The observer's role is specifically and strictly to observe how the practitioner is using the *task-centred model*, not to hypothesise about the person's situation or make general evaluative comments. By agreement, the observer can interrupt to make a suggestion if the practitioner is observed to be drifting away from the model.

BOX 4.3: EXPLORING THE PROBLEMS

Basic principle underpinning the exploring problems stage

The person's expressed and considered wishes are paramount, not the practitioner's assessment of what they 'really' want or need.
Five phases in the exploring problems phase:

1 SCAN

Looking for 'headlines'; what is the range of problems in broad shape, not specific detail. The practitioner helps to ***elicit*** the problem areas.

2 ADDITIONS

Are there any additional problems which the practitioner or others have identified and which need to be included in this picture? Are there any 'mandated problems' (by a court, for example)?
The practitioner ***discloses*** these and ***explains*** why they are important, too.

3 DETAILS

Having scanned the range of problems, each is ***investigated*** in detail, to get the 'inside story'. The investigation is a joint enterprise (i.e. not the worker investigating the user or carer, but everyone investigating each problem).

4 QUOTATIONS

Each problem area is ***summarised*** in a single statement – a direct quote using the person's own words.

5 SELECTION

The person ***prioritises*** these problems, with the aid of the practitioner, to arrive at a 'lead problem' which will be the focus of the work. Usually this is just one problem, but up to three can be selected.

Three requirements for the selected problem(s):

- The person explicitly acknowledges the problem and expresses a willingness to work on it.
- The person is in a position to take action to alleviate the problem, with the help of others such as the practitioner.
- The problem is relatively specific and limited in its scope.

Once everybody has had an opportunity to rehearse the five stages of problem exploration with a neutral case, it is important to have time for reflection. This will include making links from the neutral case to one or two current cases, to begin to move between the general and the specific. If the learners are constructing a portfolio of their learning and practice, this is an opportunity for them to have relevant pages from the portfolio to make some rough notes for themselves while the experience of the session is fresh in their minds.

The flipchart sheets are useful for many reasons, not least as a way to consider how learners can improve their use of the flipchart recording in real practice with people. Often there are one-word problem areas, with no detail, such as 'bullying' (Portfolio D 2002: 2.3). Sometimes there are interpretations:

> 'What is the problem?
> Daniel hitting [step-brother] Mat *as a way of control*.'
>
> (Portfolio D 2002: 2.3 – our italics)

ACTIVITY 4.3: TRAINER

Giving feedback from small groups to the large group

Feedback is an important aspect of most training programmes. However, there is the risk that it is repetitive and time-consuming, especially when a number of small groups have been working on the same task and are all asked to report back to each other.

- How would you organise feedback from the trios who have been rehearsing problem exploration in task-centred practice?
- What would you ask them to focus on?
- How would you avoid repetitiveness?

There is an example answer in the Appendix.

Problems confused with goals

Put simply, the problem is what is wrong and the goal is what is wanted. Possible goals are often suggested during the problem exploration stage, though these are not considered in detail until the target problem has been chosen. However, everyday use of language leads us to confuse the two: 'The problem is he thinks we should be living separate lives.' The word 'need' is especially troublesome: 'The problem is I need to move house.' Are these problems or goals? One of the teacher's aims is to ensure that people learning task-centred practice understand the differences.

Examples of problems stated as goals:

Problem areas scanned:

(i) I want to be able to choose my own drinks at home / pub / supermarket.
(ii) I want to be able to choose my own clothes with colours that look good and fabrics that feel good.

(iii) I want more recreational activities where motion is involved (e.g. fair-ground rides / train journeys).

(Portfolio I 2003: 2.2)

'I want a job, I know I can't get one, but that is what I would like.'

'I want to save some money so I need a lock-up savings tin.'

'I want to live on my own, at the seaside would be nice.'

'I want a holiday, I have never had one.'

The above were Dave's problems as he saw them.

. . . I found this stage quite difficult with Dave; he could not separate problems from wants and wishes.

(Portfolio E 2000: 2.2)

Example of a problem that might be a goal:

Problem chosen to work on:
Enrolling at college.

(Portfolio E 2000: 2.3)

Example of a goal stated as a problem:

We agreed that the cost of transport was an issue and it needed to be sorted before we could move onto his *problem of getting a job.*

(Portfolio E 2000: 2.3 – our italics)

In some senses the difference between problems and goals is semantic; a boat is as long as it is long, whatever system of measurement you use. However, if you are constructing a boat, you most definitely do need to use agreed measurements. It is in this latter respect that it is worth being particular about the differences between problems and goals, since this clarity helps everybody to understand what exactly it is that is problematic and where exactly it is that you are all going. The technique benefits from being systematic.

Avoiding the verb 'need', and beginning a statement with 'I want' or 'We want' guarantees a statement which is a goal. This is a start, but there are other factors which should be considered when finalising the goal, not least to try to arrive at a statement which is relatively clear rather than fuzzy (see Activity 4.4 and Box 4.4). Sometimes, in order to be true to a person's own words, it may be a case of recording a general statement and agreeing a second statement which indicates what will have changed to demonstrate this. For instance, a person with agoraphobic problems might have an overall, generalised goal recorded as, 'I want to be able to get out and about', with an indicator goal, such as, 'I will be able to go to the coffee bar in town on my own'.

Selecting goals

By generating ten or so examples of personal goals from the learners in the training programme, and recording these on a flipchart, it is possible to show the different qualities of various goals by asking learners to use Activity 4.4.

ACTIVITY 4.4: LEARNER

Reframing goals

Make a note of some four or five personal goals (for example, 'I want to give up smoking'). Plot your goal using the chart below.

My goal is:

Clear and specific	7 – 6 – 5 – 4 – 3 – 2 – 1	Fuzzy and general
Under my control	7 – 6 – 5 – 4 – 3 – 2 – 1	Out of my control
Involves only me	7 – 6 – 5 – 4 – 3 – 2 – 1	Involves many others
Short term	7 – 6 – 5 – 4 – 3 – 2 – 1	Long term
Time-limited	7 – 6 – 5 – 4 – 3 – 2 – 1	Open-ended
Motivating	7 – 6 – 5 – 4 – 3 – 2 – 1	Unmotivating
Easily resourced	7 – 6 – 5 – 4 – 3 – 2 – 1	Resourced with difficulty
Recently chosen	7 – 6 – 5 – 4 – 3 – 2 – 1	Long-standing
A new goal	7 – 6 – 5 – 4 – 3 – 2 – 1	A goal I've already tried

The higher the overall score, the more likelihood you have of success (maximum score: 63). Try rephrasing those goals which score relatively low so that they 'move' from right to left (i.e. achieve higher scores), while remaining faithful to the spirit of the goal.

By working on their personal goals, learners once again understand the common factors between their own personal problem-solving and goal-setting activities and those they will be using with people in their professional capacity. The task-centred method has techniques such as goal refinement which attempt to build in success while staying true to people's aspirations. In this way it is much more systematic than 'conversational' goal-setting.

Teaching task-centred practice is not just about the moving parts of the model, but very much about their relationship to one another, to the learners' current practices, and to the meaning which all those involve ascribe to these processes. This is especially true of the recorded agreement in task-centred practice. Each agreement has a common structure – a statement of the problem or problems which have been selected, a statement of the goal and a time limit, but the process of achieving the agreement is integral to a successful outcome.

BOX 4.4: SELECTING THE GOAL

Four requirements for the goal

- *Motivation*
  The person *wants* to work on this goal; it is something they actively desire to achieve, when the costs and the benefits of working towards the goal are taken into account.
- *Feasible and desirable*
  The person *can* work on this goal; it is within their capabilities, and it is one which *justifies* the worker's assistance.
- *Specific*
  There is a greater chance that a goal will be successful if it is clear rather than fuzzy, specific rather than general.
- *Related to the problem*
  It should be evident to everyone involved how success with the goal will alleviate, if not solve, the selected problem.

Examples of goals

- I want to stop smoking
- I want to sort out my financial problems
- I want to learn to play the guitar
- I want to weigh ten pounds less by the time we go on holiday in August
- We want to have a happy marriage
- I want him to help me with the housework
- I want to be rich
- I want to move from this flat by Christmas.

(Doel and Marsh 1992: 48)

Rehearsal of the process of selecting the goal and negotiating an agreement can follow the pattern established by the problem exploration workshop, with a full group demonstration by a tutor rehearsing the part of the practitioner and a volunteer playing the service user, followed by small rehearsals in threes. Familiarity with 'The Dales' from previous workshop sessions means that it is possible to move into the negotiation without too much background preparation. Possible goals can be brainstormed by the full group beforehand. Essentially, the purpose of the rehearsal is to practise helping people to frame goals which have the best likelihood of being achieved, using the criteria in Activity 4.4, linking the agreed goal to the chosen problem, and discussing the likely timescale to achieve the goal (see Box 4.5).

BOX 4.5: NEGOTIATING THE AGREEMENT

Three elements to the agreement

- the selected problem(s)
- the goal(s)
- the time limit and frequency of contact.

Time limits: 'from headlines to deadlines'

The time limit is a brief statement about the likely length of time needed to reach the goal. This is an estimate, decided in discussion between all the parties to the discussion.

Yardstick

The time limit is important to provide the yardstick by which progress will be measured (one-quarter the way to our time limit; nearly two-thirds through, etc.). It helps to focus the efforts of everybody involved and accelerates these efforts. The time limit should feel near enough to have an impact.

Frequency

In addition to the time limit, an agreement should be made about the likely frequency of contact during the period. This provides a kind of map for everybody involved.

Developing and reviewing tasks

The practice of developing and reviewing tasks and the use of a sequence known as Task Planning and Implementation is described in Chapter 3 and illustrated in Chapter 6. In this chapter we will concern ourselves with issues arising from teaching these elements in the model. Boxes 4.6, 4.7, 4.8 and 4.9 can be used as handouts to support teaching task development, implementation and review.

One of the benefits of continuing with 'The Dales' as the principal case example is the learners' familiarity with their circumstances. However, in terms of process, some variety can be achieved by suggesting that workshop participants might like to take turns in the practitioner 'hot seat' to rehearse in the full group, rather than breaking into threes (as they did for earlier rehearsals of the method). Much will depend on the confidence of the group members, but this is a good opportunity for direct feedback to several individuals in turn, and for everyone to witness the variety of styles which can be used, even with the same basic structure. The person playing the service user (usually 'Janet Dale') should be changed from time to time, so that no single person feels 'locked' into the role. Rehearsals are best stopped after five or so minutes, so that the review can be focused and fresh (it becomes increasingly hard to remember the detail of an exchange as time goes on). The person rehearsing the practitioner's part needs to know that they can bring proceedings to a halt whenever they wish. Feedback should be given along the lines of 'What would you keep, what would you change?' rather than evaluative feeback of the 'What went well, what didn't go so well?' nature. Particularly productive questions to ask the full group are 'What alternatives might have been taken?' and 'How would you advise we should proceed from here?'. This spreads the responsibility for the rehearsal out from the individual playing the practitioner's role to the whole group.

The task planning and implementation sequence needs to be detailed and discussed so that everyone knows what it consists of and why it is important. Participants can then break into small groups to practise this technique. Another variant of the rehearsal at this stage is to introduce task-centred work with couples or families, with the suggestion that people break into slightly larger groups of four or five, rehearsing with both Janet and John Dale or Janet Dale and her mother-in-law, Jean Dale, for instance. Starting the process with the simplest formation (a practitioner and one individual) makes sense, but by this stage participants should have more confidence with the model and with each other to consider more complex structures, which could also involve two practitioners.

The rehearsals enable learners to make some common mistakes, such as assuming that a 'ladder of tasks' needs to be planned for the whole sequence of work, from start to finish, rather than the tasks evolving stage by stage as the work unfolds. These are often best learnt through the experience of rehearsal rather than being 'told' by the course teachers.

The rehearsals of task review should contain an instance of a task that has largely been successful and one which has not been achieved. This provides an opportunity to rehearse how to look for learning from both kinds of experience and to discover how unsuccessful tasks can still achieve successful learning. Learners often feel uncomfortable with the rating system for task achievement, yet the experiences recorded in portfolios of task-centred practice suggest that the rating system is very valuable. One of the points of rehearsal is to practise, and repeatedly practise, new techniques which might at first feel unfamiliar, even uncomfortable; some people will throw themselves into these new experiences and others will need coaxing.

As with the rehearsals of the earlier stages of task-centred practice, participants should become familiar with using flipchart paper as an integral part of the process of developing options for tasks, using the task sequence and reviewing task achievement (see Boxes 4.6 to 4.9).

Evaluating the work together

The final element of the programme is evaluating the task-centred work. Participants in a workshop can be asked to consider how they currently evaluate their work with people and to identify for themselves areas of practice which they would wish to keep, and areas they would wish to change and develop. Students who may not have any direct professional practice to draw on can be asked to consider themselves as users of a service, the more recent the better (such as using a dentist, a transport service, a bank, a plumber, etc.), and to evaluate that service in terms of its outcome for them, and also the process. It is possible, for example, to have visited a dentist and had the pain relieved (successful outcome), while feeling dissatisfied with the dentist's manner and treatment of you (unsuccessful process). Alternatively, you may be very happy with the way the dentist treated you as a person (successful process), yet still be in some pain (unsuccessful outcome).

BOX 4.6: DEVELOPING TASKS

Tasks are the actions which help people to move from the problem to the goal. Tasks help everyone to put the problem-solving plan into operation. They should build from one session to another, so that the successful completion of tasks by Session A helps to develop further tasks to complete by Session B.

Different types of task

- Session tasks *completed during the session itself*
- Homework tasks *completed between sessions*
- Unique tasks
- Recurrent tasks
- Individual tasks *(J will . . .)*
- Reciprocal tasks *(J will . . . and K will . . .)*
- Shared tasks *(J and K will . . .)*

A checklist

What should be done:

- Have you found out what has worked in the past?
- Have you worked co-operatively together to produce the suggested task?
- Will the task help the progress towards the goal?
- Is there a reasonable balance between practitioner tasks and service user and carer tasks?

Why this task?

- Do people understand the reason for the task and how it moves towards the goal?
- How were 'inappropriate' suggestions for tasks handled?
- Was a positive expectation about the chances of success conveyed?
- Are people motivated to attempt their tasks?

How a task should be done:

- Is the task specific enough for you all to know how successful it will have been?
- Have you all anticipated possible difficulties?
- Has 'coaching' for the task taken place where appropriate and necessary?
- Is everyone clear that progress will be reviewed at the next session, and when this is?

BOX 4.7: TASK PLANNING AND IMPLEMENTATION SEQUENCE

The Task Planning and Implementation Sequence (TPIS) is a series of steps to be carried out flexibly to help task achievement.

Reid (1975, 1992, 2000) found clear improvements in the completion of tasks when this kind of sequence was followed.

There are seven elements to the TPIS:

- *Task selection*
  What do you think you might be able to do about this problem? Generate options.
- *Task agreement*
  This is reached after alternative possibilities have been sorted out and the best selected.
- *Planning specifics of implementation*
  Once a task is selected, a plan is developed; tasks that have been borrowed from *The Task Planner* (Reid 2000) need customising.
- *Establishing incentives and rationale*
  What might you gain from doing this task?
- *Anticipating obstacles*
  'What if?' questions help people to think about how the task could fail.
- *Simulated and guided practice*
  Modelling and rehearsal; or accompanying a person in a real-life situation.

At the next session:

- *Task review*
  Reviewing progress on the task (usually at the next session) is a crucial element in task implementation. This involves everyone learning from the experience, whether the task was relatively successful or not.

BOX 4.8: TPIS IN PRACTICE

See Activity 4.2 for the background to Janet Dale's situation.

Selected problem

- Janet finds it difficult to do things with the children. For example, 'I don't have the confidence to bath them'.

Agreed goal

- 'I [Janet] want to feel confident bathing the children.'

Directly involved in this goal are Janet, Jean and the children, with help from John and the social worker.

Time limit

- Six weeks; contact once a week for six weeks.

Given the selected problem as:

> 'I [Janet] find it difficult to do things with the children. For example, I don't have the confidence to bath them.'

use the TPIS to help the family develop the first tasks towards resolving this problem.

Suggested process

In small groups, rehearse the TPIS by allocating roles of social worker, Janet, Jean, observer(s). Use the TPIS to select and implement two tasks.

The observer's comments should be focused solely around the way in which the social worker is following the sequence.

Make a note on flipchart paper of headlines which summarise the way the sequence has been used. Move on to the task review (i.e. the next session) if you have time; rehearse one task which was successful and one which was not.

BOX 4.9: REVIEWING TASKS

After the agreement has been negotiated and written down, each session will include a period in which the tasks agreed at the previous session are discussed and reviewed, followed by a period when new tasks are developed. These tasks will, in turn, be reviewed at the following session, etc.

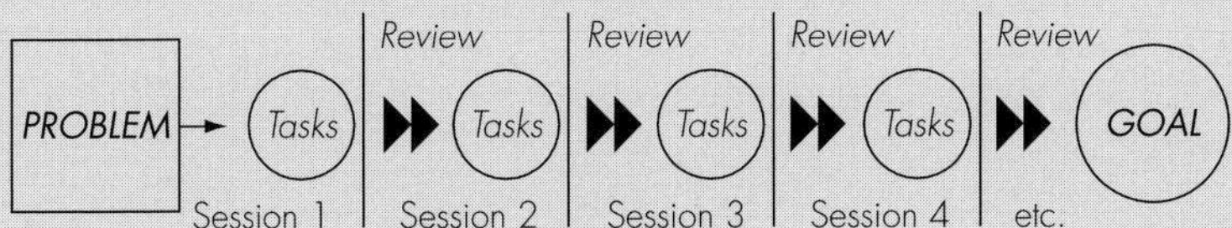

Progress to goal

The review of tasks is an important opportunity to check on the progress towards the goal. Each set of tasks should move nearer to the achievement of the goal; achieving the tasks will be a visible sign of movement towards the goal.

Learning from tasks – successful or not

There should be positive encouragement for successful tasks, with some discussion about how easy or difficult the task was. Tasks which were unsuccessful, or only partially completed need to be analysed carefully, looking at obstacles, how they were dealt with and what can be learned from this. Often, more can be learned from unsuccessful tasks than from successful ones, so it is important not to lose this opportunity, either by attributing blame or by glossing over difficulties in a mistaken attempt to minimise the lack of success.

The difference between process and outcome is a useful distinction and forms the basis of the questions which practitioners will be using with people at the end of the task-centred work. Box 4.10 can serve as a handout and a cribsheet for practice. Once again, it is important to rehearse this part of the model to gain some familiarity with it before using it in direct practice (see Activities 4.5 and 4.6).

BOX 4.10: EVALUATING THE WORK TOGETHER

The final session reviews the progress that has been made towards achieving the goal. However, in addition to this, it is a good opportunity to review and evaluate all your work together and a chance to give useful feedback and encouragement for the future.

Suggested questions to ask at the final session

These questions are asked because I would like you to let me know what you think about the work we have done together, and to help me to improve my work. This will help us both to get the best out of the ending of our work.

- *The beginning*
  Looking back to the beginning of our work, why do you think I got involved with you?
- *The problem*
  Do you think the problem that you chose to work on was the right one? How has the problem changed? Has it got better?
- *Our written agreement*
  What did you think about our written agreement? Did you like this style of work? For example, did it help to use pens and paper in our work together?
- *The goal*
  How near to your goal are you? What tells you how near you are to your goal? How near to your goal do other people think you are?
- *In general*
  Looking over the work we have done together, what was most useful? What was least useful – how might we have done some things differently?
- *The future*
  Now that we have finished our work together, will you try this way of doing things without me? What will you need to make it successful?

ACTIVITY 4.5: SERVICE USER OR CARER

Contributing to the teaching of task-centred practice

In addition to your feedback on the experience of using task-centred practice (see Box 4.10), how else could you see yourself contributing to the ways in which this method of practice is taught?

ACTIVITY 4.6: MANAGER

Improving the flow of information in the agency

- The evaluations of task-centred work (Box 4.10) provide much valuable information. While ensuring proper confidentiality for the individuals concerned, how might this information be collated to improve the quality of services which the agency provides?
- How might the information from evaluations of task-centred work (Box 4.10) be used to inform the agency's policy and practice on continuing professional development?

PUTTING IT ALL INTO PRACTICE

In an agency-based training course, it is beneficial to have two consecutive days of workshops in which the whole of the method can be taught in a sequence which takes participants from the beginning to end of the method. Preparation in the form of consultations with paired participants and their supervisors beforehand is likely to improve understanding and follow-through (see Box 4.1). A gap of about three weeks between this workshop and a further one-hour consultation enables participants to start to practise the method with real people and to use the consultation to raise issues arising from this experience.

Further workshops allow participants to learn from one another's experiences and provide mutual support for the extra effort needed to sustain a new practice method. The workshop and consultation dates are useful deadlines for learners to work towards, all of which mirror the use of motivational time limits in the task-centred work itself.

A 'buddy' system, in which pairs of practitioners support each other through the training programme, is likely to encourage the transfer of learning from the workshop or classroom into direct practice, especially if the pair have the chance to work together on a task-centred sequence of work. Compiling a portfolio of task-centred work is also likely to reinforce the learning and to encourage continuing reflection on the professional development. All of these extra reinforcements are important, since the pressure to slip back into pre-workshop styles and patterns of work is very great (Marsh and Triseliotis 1996; Rushton and Martyn 1990). The support and direction of the supervisor or line manager is significant in helping practitioners to sustain the changes that they have made, so some involvement of supervisors in the training programme brings much benefit. A supervisor who makes the time to join the consultations with the tutors in effect becomes a part of the teaching team. Though the supervisor's knowledge of the task-centred method is unlikely to be as detailed as the practitioner who has completed a full training programme, the supervisor's role in providing encouragement and space can be crucial (Activity 4.7).

ACTIVITY 4.7: SUPERVISOR

Sustaining the work

What might your role be in the teaching team which is helping practitioners to learn the task-centred method and to put it into practice?

What is likely to help the task-centred work?	What might hinder it?
OPPORTUNITIES	OBSTACLES

What difference does the teaching make?

There is a daunting number of variables in the relationship between the teaching of task-centred practice and changes in the lives of people engaged in task-centred work. What additional benefit, if any, does a taught programme have over, say, reading this book? What elements in a taught programme are most effective (The rehearsals? The consultations? Having the support of a supervisor? Participating with a paired practitioner? Being in a paired arrangement?) and how does this vary from one person to another? The variables are also enormous when we consider the technology of the method of practice. Is it important to have a clear distinction in the language between problems and goals? Does a recorded agreement (as opposed to a verbal one) make a difference to the outcome? What is the optimum time limit for what kinds of goal? Do agreements with individuals have any different success rate than those made with more than one person?

Task-centred practice is relatively well researched, with a tried and tested collection of 'task planners' (Reid 2000), but the complexity of practice means we must be tentative about answers to the questions just posed. The portfolios of task-centred practice which we have used extensively to illustrate this book are a valuable window on the relationship between teaching, learning and practice. They draw heavily on self-report, but they regularly demonstrate an honesty and authenticity which suggests they provide reliable insights into the difference which task-centred practice has made both to the lives of service users and carers and to the professional competence and satisfaction of the workers.

One social care worker, who did not hold a professional qualification, expressed three notable changes 'before and after'. The first concerns the way she and the team had been working with people; the second is in respect of her own role in the team; and the third relates to her own developing perspective on task-centred practice:

> We aim to help clients with issues but these tend not to be client-selected problems, but problems the practitioner feels will be the most beneficial to focus upon.
>
> In the past I have been briefed by qualified members of staff regarding my role in the work with a client, rather than determining what the client actually wants.
>
> Many believe that they use the task-centred approach by simply carrying out tasks rather than taking into consideration all other aspects of the practice. The approach has the image of being brisk but the reality is that it is a complex practice, which involves theory as well as practicality.
>
> (Portfolio K 2002: 2.3; 1.4)

Task-centred practice is an educational model of practice

In essence, a task-centred intervention is a series of workshops to teach problem-solving. Task-centred practice is at its most effective when service users and carers understand the *workings* of the model, over and above the specific application of the model to meet their circumstances. The practitioner's role is as much teacher as any other, and the theoretical basis of the task-centred practice draws on learning and educational theory more than any other. The use of specific techniques, especially flipcharting, reinforces a sense of the session as a workshop rather than a meeting or interview.

This sense of task-centred practice as an adult education course in life skills and problem-solving is reinforced by the links which are repeatedly made between this method of professional practice and the personal problem-solving, goal-achieving activities which are a common aspect of most if not all people's lives. For example, one practitioner recorded how she had taught a colleague the method:

> In addition to making use of the task planning and implementation sequence in my professional practice, I have explored the use of this in my personal life. A colleague is undertaking a university course which is becoming a heavy burden and she was considering pulling out of the course despite her strong desire to achieve her qualifications. We used the Task Planning and Implementation Sequence in order to motivate her and equip her with the skills needed to complete the course.
>
> (Portfolio F 2003: 4.2)

In addition to direct practice with people, task-centred principles have been adapted to develop a method of supervision for staff and students in social work and related professions. Task-centred supervision (TCS) is an educational model which contrasts with therapeutic (and, indeed managerial) approaches 'in that it emphasizes a discovery of alternative interpersonal actions instead of an examination of intrapsychic or family-of-origin "issues"' (Caspi and Reid 2002: 104). Once again, it is the educational potential of the task-centred method which is prominent.

KEY POINTS

- ☐ The training programme should be structured to enable participants to use the task-centred method with at least one user or carer during the course of the programme.
- ☐ The involvement of the participants' line manager is crucial to deliver the support necessary to put the learning into practice.
- ☐ Paired participants are able to reinforce one another's learning when the workshop ends and the real practice begins.
- ☐ It is important to engage with people's different notions of causality, because these influence their practices and worldviews.
- ☐ It is important to teach the difference between problems and goals.
- ☐ Compiling an assessed portfolio helps to reinforce the teaching and learning.

KEY READING

Caspi, J. and Reid, W. J. (2002) *Educational Supervision in Social Work: A Task-centred Model for Field Instruction and Staff Development* New York: Columbia University Press

This gives a useful account of how the task-centred practice model can be transferred to staff development, in the supervision of either staff or students.

Stepney, P. and Ford, D. (2000) *Social Work Models, Methods and Theories: A Framework for Practice* Lyme Regis, UK: Russel House

This is a useful general guide to the distinctions between different methods, and also between the notions of models, methods and theories.

Schön, D. (1987) *Educating the Reflective Practitioner* San Francisco, CA: Josey-Bass

This is a few years old, but it remains a classic in terms of teaching and learning processes in professional practice; it is especially interesting because it considers a range of professions beyond health and social care.

See also Key Reading for Chapter 8.

CHAPTER 5

LEARN

OBJECTIVES

By the end of this chapter you should:

- Understand the key issues in learning the task-centred model
- Appreciate possible barriers to learning and the emotional impact of learning
- Challenge assumptions and engage in 'unlearning'
- Reflect on learning and practice using 'prompts'
- Know how evidence of learning can be gathered and demonstrated.

STARTING WHERE THE LEARNER IS

Though learning is an everyday experience, it is nevertheless an exciting process. (We will use the term 'learner' to denote anybody who is learning about task-centred practice; this is a more inclusive term than 'students' [which, in the UK, usually means people who are not yet qualified] and 'candidates' [used solely for people who are studying for post-qualification and post-registration awards]. 'Learner' also includes people who are not enrolled in any formal programme of study and, of course, it can encompass people who learn about task-centred practice as service users or carers.) There is still much to discover about the transfer from 'learning about' to 'learning to do', and how to convert learning in simulated or class-based settings into practical changes in professional practice (Cree and Macaulay 2000). The purpose and context of learning are significant in this process, especially an awareness of possible barriers and blocks.

Learning often focuses on the development of new skills and abilities (such as learning to drive a car), yet the success of new learning owes much to the way in which it can adapt to the current meanings which the particular learner attributes to this experience. Learners' past experiences of the world have shaped their current understanding of it, and it is important to acknowledge this if the challenge of new learning is to be meaningful and acceptable. Sometimes this means trying to find the relationship between different terminologies. For example, the need to avoid 'becoming solutional', a tendency to offer solutions during the problem exploration stage of task-centred practice, might be understood in postmodernist terms as 'facilitating the narrative', asking illuminating questions rather than giving answers as an expert (Dean 1998). Both processes are very similar, but the language does not make this obvious and could be a barrier to learning.

It is, therefore, important to relate task-centred principles and practices to the learners' existing values and ways of working. In what ways have learners used problem-solving methods before, either in their professional or personal life?

> On reflection I can recognise elements of my previous practice that bore resemblance to the task centred model, [such as a] clear mandate, time-limited intervention, realistic goal setting and regular reviewing.
>
> (Portfolio F 2003: 2.1)

We approach new situations by considering how they relate to what we already know and how we already do things. In order to accept the challenge implicit in the learning of different practice, we need to know why and how these differences are desirable and to feel that our current strengths are appreciated.

Unlearning

One of the strengths of the task-centred model is the ease with which it fits most practitioners' existing values and practices. Most learners feel that their practice is founded on principles of openness and partnership, and that their work involves tasks to help to achieve certain outcomes. Paradoxically, this supposed fit is also a major disadvantage. The sense of 'doing all that already' (Marsh 1990) can block the unlearning which is needed to translate the idea of working in partnership into reality (see 'The Dales' exercise in Chapter 4). Fixed ideas, for example, about what a 'task' is and what constitutes an 'agreement', can inhibit new practices. It is similar to the way experienced two-finger typists must unlearn some of their existing typing techniques in order to achieve a better level of typing.

One practitioner describes 'biting her tongue' in order to prevent herself from slipping into the groove of a well-worn pattern of working:

> During both the problem scans [in two separate pieces of task-centred work] I felt that I was constantly biting my tongue to stop myself being solutional . . . I think I managed well not to offer solutions, probably because I had anticipated this. I wonder whether this will feel easier in time?
>
> (Portfolio J 2002: 2.2)

Another relatively experienced worker reflects on the difference between old and new practices:

> In a 'normal' piece of work with a new client . . . I would be more concerned with team 'wants' and statutory 'wants', regardless that they were not [service user or carer] 'needs'.
>
> (Portfolio B 2002: 2.3)

Being conscious of the ways in which the learning is affecting the practice is part of the learning itself. If it does not *feel* different, then it is not different. The practice of using people's own quotations is something which the following practitioner had learned about in theory in a workshop, but came to know the value in practice by trying something new.

> Writing down what Wayne was saying was useful in two ways. First I was able to keep it in his own words. Even when you repeat back to a service user what they have said you can alter the meaning slightly. But putting it on paper for both of us to see helped to stop this. Secondly, using this way of recording allowed me to be both systematic and responsive. For example, because something had been written down it was easy to come back to it if we wandered off the track slightly, as can often happen.
>
> (Portfolio F 2003: 2.2)

It may be necessary to unlearn some preconceptions about what task-centred practice is. The term 'task-centred' can be confusing, since it seems to suggest that relationships and feelings are relegated to the all-important doing of tasks. As we explained in Chapter 3, tasks do play a central part in the effectiveness of the model, but this way of working is as person-centred as any other method of work with users and carers, perhaps much more so. It is a highly reflective practice which focuses on tasks only in so far as they can help *people*:

> Task-centred practice has made me more aware of how intricate and problematic relationships can be in families . . . I will incorporate into more of my practice looking at the broader canvas of problems within families and not just at what has been identified on the referral.
>
> (Portfolio D 2002: 2.3)

It can be important to unlearn the service user's past, too. One service user, John, had a reputation as having problems with female workers, but the (female) task-centred practitioner records a quite different experience in her task-centred portfolio:

> Recordings have shown in the past that John has had trouble engaging with female members of staff. John's lack of engagement was due to him having deluded ideas, regarding women being the 'spawn of the devil'. These perceptions cannot be linked to any known or recorded instances. I am unsure whether John has any feelings regarding power and oppression with women, as the only experience I have had with John contradicts his past ideas as he stated, 'I can tell you have been sent from God!'.
>
> (Portfolio K 2002: 2)

Since past and present workers were women, the gender of the practitioner seems to be less of a factor than whether John felt he was being listened to.

Eclectic practice

There is in social work a sense that reliance on a particular theory or method is constraining, almost unnatural. The work is so varied and needs such flexible responses that no single model could possibly suit all situations, so it is with some pride that most practitioners declare themselves 'eclectic'. We suspect this is common to other professions, too. The worker below reflects this unease:

> Throughout my early years as a social worker I drew from my knowledge of different theories and did not depend on one theory. I never felt comfortable relying on one theory as I found that I did not always agree with all aspects of all theories. I mixed and matched the parts I felt were appropriate and worked for me. I find that I still practise like this today. I do not follow the [solution-focused therapy] model religiously, as there are aspects of it that I feel uncomfortable with, in particular the miracle question. Reflecting on the work that I have done so far, it is the timing of the model that I have altered and in some cases I have missed out using the miracle question.
>
> (General [PQ1] portfolio 2003, Critical Career Review)

It is difficult to know whether the question of eclecticism is, indeed, a careful decision not to be bound to any particular theory, and to refuse to adhere to a specific model. A true eclecticism is built on a sound understanding of a number of different methods and an appreciation of what works best in which circumstances, based on prolonged experience of these different methods. However, there is also the possibility that an approach that is called eclectic is one which provides a rationale for practice which has been learnt ad hoc rather than in any systematic fashion, with patterns of practice determined by existing gridlines which themselves have been etched in haphazard ways. If this latter explanation is near the mark, it is likely that there will be a need for considerable 'unlearning', and that this will prove especially challenging. The badge of eclecticism can be a barrier to learning the task-centred method (see Activity 5.1).

ACTIVITY 5.1: PRACTITIONER

Challenges to learning the task-centred model

George is a social worker who has been qualified for over fifteen years. He is in sympathy with the values and principles of task-centred practice and claims that he has been using a task-centred 'approach' in much of his work. However, he has never used an agreement, does not record the work in the way he has been learning in the task-centred workshops, and has never formally evaluated his work with a service user.

What do you think are the major challenges that George will face as he learns the task-centred model?

THE SHOCK OF THE NEW

Learning is as much an emotional experience as it is a cognitive one (Eraut 2004).

> Learning means adapting to change and finding ways to access specialist discourses and practices. This can lead to uncertainty, disorientation and feelings of powerlessness and loss of status or identity.
>
> (Atkins 2002: 61)

It can also be exciting, even exhilarating. Putting the learning from task-centred workshops into actual practice can feel much more challenging and different than learners anticipate. The willingness to unlearn some established patterns, or at least to work in ways which might feel uncomfortable because they are different, is crucial to sustain the learning into regular practice. If learners know that they may feel deskilled initially as they try new techniques, this will help them to remain committed to the effort which is needed. For students this kind of new experience is expected, but experienced practitioners need particular support from supervisors and team members if they are to find emotional and practical space to maintain these changes.

The task-centred work can provide a significantly new kind of experience for the service user and carer, too. In their contact with the various services, people learn about them and are shaped by them. If task-centred practice can give people a positive experience of professional contact, this can have wider consequences.

> I strongly believe that this stage of work was very empowering for Kelly. Having never been consulted during past experiences with mental health services she has always been told what is wrong with her, where she should live and how she should manage her difficulties and, therefore, has always been placed in a position where she did not feel listened to or understood.
>
> (Portfolio B 2002: 3)

Task-centred work can help people to develop new ways of thinking about themselves – 'new narratives', to use the postmodern jargon. This can help to undo some of the established truths which people have learned to accept about themselves, and produce what Howard (1991) has called 'story repair'. However, learning requires us to take risks by moving a certain distance outside our zone of comfort and if this is too far, we can become defensive and learning becomes frozen (see Activity 5.2). The use of video, with informed consent, to capture the task-centred work was a step too far for this practitioner and the service user:

> If absolutely honest, I felt totally uncomfortable with the idea of being filmed and was more than pleased when Wayne failed to arrive for our session!
>
> (Portfolio F 2003: 7.1)

ACTIVITY 5.2: TRAINER

A workshop on task-centred practice for learners

You are invited to run a series of workshops on task-centred practice with a group of twelve learners in the same agency. Some participants are qualified practitioners and very experienced, some are newly qualified and some are pre-qualified.

- What do you anticipate might be some of the main issues for this group of learners?
- How could you encourage learners to 'unlearn' some elements of their current practice?
- What might hinder and what might help the group's learning and practice of task-centred work?
- How will you take account of the emotional dimension of learning?

When the penny drops

> I had thought that Task A was self-explanatory and although I understood the process of the Task Planning and Implementation Sequence, I don't think I had fully understood or appreciated its purpose, though I didn't realise this until Sharon and I actually went through the process . . . or, in colloquial terms, 'the penny dropped' for me.
>
> (Portfolio A 2000: 4.2)

The experience of this practitioner illustrates the complexity of 'learning how to . . .', and how this is different from 'knowledge of . . .'. Part of the complexity is that we may not even be aware that our understanding is lacking until we put it into practice, like the clothes on the hanger that look as though they fit, but are too short when we put them on.

There are strong parallels between the learning for the practitioner (and supervisor) and the learning for service users and carers. For many people the experience of task-centred practice is very new; to have a person who focuses on your problems and what you want, who gives time and attention to the details in your life, who shows understanding and commitment to helping you make a success, all of this can be a radical departure from past experiences. Some tasks may require a person to consider or do something which is starkly different from their past habit:

> On the surface, this [task] appears to be a very simplistic thing to do, as many people walk away from conflict. Wayne had never experienced doing this and usually jumped in feet first. Wayne said that he felt 'great' when he was able to walk away from his sister's argument and he described 'rising above it'.
>
> (Portfolio F 2003: 4.3)

Just as the penny sometimes takes a while to drop for the practitioner, so too for the service user or carer. Learning and the changes which it brings can be a mix of exhilaration and fear. Learning about something of which you were not previously aware, making something explicit and open which has been implicit and hidden, learning to do something which you have not considered yourself able to do, all of this involves risk. For

Wayne, the process of putting into writing his problems and his goals made them very real and he described this as 'scary', as this made him 'face up' to reality (Portfolio F 2003: 3.1).

Perhaps most shocking of all is learning to be someone you have not seen yourself to be (or others have not seen you to be). Overcoming the internalised self as someone who is bad, stupid, clumsy, etc., takes the most risk and the most courage.

> It was critical, at this stage, to encourage Kelly to acknowledge that having problems were not a reflection on her being 'stupid' or 'useless', but were as a result of her childhood experiences and mental ill health. Rather that she was showing strength and determination in taking control of her situation and attempting to change it.
>
> (Portfolio B 2002: 2.2)

These changes in self-image may not occur with the suddenness of a penny dropping, but are more likely to be part of a longer process, more like layers of a veil being removed one by one. This process of unveiling may well be incomplete by the end of the work with the practitioner, but the task-centred method is designed so that people can learn how to continue the unveiling themselves, independent of the worker. Learning how the veil was gathered in the first place, through processes of oppression and discrimination at social and personal levels, may be an important aspect of the person's learning. However, it may also be possible to experience these changes in self-definition without this analysis, much as it is possible to learn how to untangle a ball of wool without knowing how or why it first became tangled. Together with the service users and carers, the task-centred practitioner must make that judgement (see Activity 5.3).

ACTIVITY 5.3: SERVICE USER AND CARER

Learning a new skill, behaviour or attitude

Think of a new skill, behaviour or attitude you have learned, or a new situation you have learned to manage.

- What changes were necessary as part of the learning?
- What helped, or would have helped, to promote these changes?
- What hindered, or might have hindered, these changes?

Challenging worldviews

It should now be evident that task-centred practice involves learning and that learning involves risk and challenge. Although these risks are taken by workers, service users and carers together, it is the service users and carers who face the greatest challenge. The practitioner's challenge is often to consider to what extent to respect the user's current view of the world and to what extent to confront it. The task-centred method ensures that workers are open to having their own worldviews challenged by service users and carers. A worker describes how she felt uncertain about whether and how to challenge the service user's own definition. What the worker saw as 'illness' the service user, John, saw as 'problem':

> It was difficult for me to contribute one of the additional problems – I felt discussing John's lack of compliance with medication was difficult, as in some respects I knew I was challenging John's beliefs about the concept of *illness* versus *problem*. . . . It was difficult for me to overcome the feelings of embarrassment, lack of experience in the model as well as being an unqualified member of staff. The newness of mine and John's relationship hindered us slightly in that I was unsure of how far I could take issues without causing offence.
>
> (Portfolio K 2002: 2.2 – our emphasis)

This is an example of how the specific use of the 'additional problems' technique is helpful (see Chapters 2 and 6 for more detail). In the preamble to the problem scan it is important to refer to the possibility of the worker adding problems as he or she sees them; something like, 'We'll consider all the problems you're experiencing, and it may be that there will be some problems that I will want to raise, too'. This prepares the ground for the worker's perceptions to be shared, as well. 'Do you remember we agreed that I would also add any problems which I can see, if they are not ones which you have identified? These are no more or no less important than those you have identified, but they are part of the picture.'

Another worker came to realise that 'what I felt passed for independent living skills and what Dan felt passed for independent living skills may well have been completely different' (Portfolio L 2000: 2.1).

LEARNING FROM REFLECTION

People consolidate their learning as they undertake agreed tasks and review progress on them with the worker. Practitioners and students can take their learning a step further by reflecting on their use of the task-centred method, either in a reflective diary or as part of a portfolio of their work. The quotations from portfolios which illustrate this book demonstrate how important it is to spend time reflecting and writing about practice. This is true of all professional practice, not just task-centred work (Doel *et al.* 2002; Yelloly and Henkel 1995). The task-centred portfolio is constructed with regular sections to encourage reflection (Doel and Marsh 1995), each introduced by a prompt (see Box 5.1).

Two practitioners reflected on how they introduced the task-centred model to the service user. Although their reflections are very different, there is clear evidence of learning in both statements.

> If this stage of the work could be revisited, I would approach the explanation of the work differently. I felt the need to go into long and explicit detail about the work, probably for my own clarification. The family had a clear agenda, and were not in the best frame of mind for listening. A more simplified, short explanation would have been more effective.
>
> (Portfolio D 2002: 2.2)

> When Sharon had referred herself to the Pre–5s Centre for a programme of work, I didn't explain that we were going to use the task-centred model, despite having the opportunity to do so. The reasons I gave myself at the time were that:

> (1) *Any* method used with Sharon would be new to her, never having worked with the Centre before, so I didn't feel a need to explain this particular one. (I realised later that this defeats the whole underpinning principles of task-centred practice.)
> (2) That Sharon would somehow lose confidence in my ability as a worker if she thought I wasn't completely *au fait* with the method we were using.
>
> However, having reached the end of this entire piece of task-centred work, and taking much opportunity to reflect, I think reason (2) was more about how able I felt at this time to share the balance of power with Sharon, and needing to appear to be 'the expert'. One of the factors influencing this may have been the knowledge that Sharon has worked as a teacher, and I have worked as a nursery-nurse. Had we both been sharing a workplace setting, Sharon would effectively have been my 'boss'. I think this contributed to me initially finding it difficult to admit that I had never used the task-centred method before. It's interesting to note that as I truly began to understand the principles of task-centred practice, it became very easy to learn together and not present myself as 'the expert'.
>
> (Portfolio A 2000: 6.1)

What strikes the reader is not the initial mistakes, but the practitioners' openness to learning by reflecting honestly on their practice. Clearly, these are workers who are very open to reflecting on their own practice, but there seems to be evidence from the full range of portfolios that the task-centred method has a positive impact on the worker's openness, not just with the service user, but with themselves. This honesty draws dividends when it brings service users, carers and practitioners together, all as learners.

> I reassured [the service user] that this was the first time I had used this method and that he in fact was helping me.
>
> (Portfolio E 2000: 3)

This approach really does begin to equalise the power between people. This levelling effect is reinforced by the fact that, as a problem-solving model, task-centred work has much in common with the ways in which we can all take more control of our lives, whether we are service users, carers, workers, or indeed all of these roles in different circumstances. As one worker noted, 'Life experience has taught me that I flourish when I form realistic aspirations, rather than wanting the unachievable' (Portfolio B 2002: 3.1).

It is often said, with much irony, that hindsight is a wonderful thing. It is true that hindsight can be used to justify or defend past actions and provide post hoc rationalisations. However, the portfolio makes frequent and positive use of the notion of hindsight by asking people to use the distance between then and now to reconsider rather than to rationalise their actions (see Activity 5.4).

> With hindsight, I would have involved Sue, Wayne's mother, to a greater degree. Ultimately, when the task-centred work ceases, the service user is left in their original home environment and often will rely on family members for support or assistance in making changes in their lives.
>
> (Portfolio F 2003: 5.2)

> Next time I begin a Scanning for Problems session I won't begin with 'How have things been?'; I'll explain the process and go a step at a time.
>
> (Portfolio A 2000: 2.2)

BOX 5.1: REFLECTIVE LEARNING

Examples of prompts in the reflective sections of the task-centred portfolio

- Consider what you have learned about your practice at this stage in the work. What similarities and what differences are there between your task-centred work and your other work? *[2.1 Mandate for involvement]*
- If you could revisit this stage in the intervention, what might you do differently and why? *[2.2 Scanning problems]*
- What have you learned about your own practice from this stage in the task-centred model? What do you most want to incorporate into your regular professional practice? *[2.3 Selecting a problem]*
- Task-centred practice is a problem-solving, goal-oriented way of working. In what ways is this similar or different to the approach which you take to your own life and/or work problems and aspirations? *[3.1 Negotiating the written agreement]*
- On reflection, what other tasks could you have developed with the service users and carers which might have achieved the same ends? *[4.1 Developing tasks]*
- How do you see yourself developing the TPIS sequence in your future task-centred practice? *[4.2 Task Planning and Implementation Sequence]*
- What do you consider are the purposes of reviewing tasks? What have you learned from the experience of reviewing tasks with the service users and carers? *[4.3 Reviewing tasks]*
- What learning have you gained from the experience of evaluating the task-centred intervention together with the service users and carers? *[5.1 Evaluation – the outcome]*
- With hindsight, what parts of the process would you keep and what might you do differently? *[5.2 Evaluation – the process]*
- With hindsight, would you make any changes to the way you recorded the task-centred work (what and why)? What have you learned from this method of recording, and what kind of impact has it had in your regular recording, if any? *[5.3 Evaluation – recording task-centred practice]*
- [You earlier described two incidents which illustrated an issue of power and oppression in your task-centred work]. Using one of these two examples, speculate on how different the experience might have been if your gender, race, sexuality, disability, etc. had been different (choose two differences). What kind of impact do you think this might have had on the work? *[6 Power and oppression]*
- Rewrite a section of dialogue to show, with hindsight, what you would change. *[7.1 Video extract]*

(Doel and Marsh 1995)

ACTIVITY 5.4: SUPERVISOR

Encouraging a multidisciplinary team to become learners

Katya is a team leader supervising ten practitioners in a multidisciplinary team. One of the practitioners is completing a post-qualifying course in task-centred practice. Another worker in the team is about to supervise a student who would like to learn how to use task-centred practice. Katya would like to encourage the whole team to become learners and sees task-centred practice as one way to facilitate this.

- What might the main issues be for Katya and the team?
- How might she encourage the whole team to 'become learners'?
- How could the questions in Box 5.1 be enlisted to help transfer and widen the task-centred learning throughout the team?

EVIDENCE OF LEARNING

How do you know whether the learning is effective, and in what ways can this be measured? Clearly, the task-centred portfolio is a significant record of learning, but not everybody who practises task-centred work has access to a portfolio. Fortunately, the task-centred model has 'built-in' mechanisms to encourage this process of measurement. The fact that the work is recorded in a carefully structured way means that practitioners have access to a regular account of their work (see Chapters 6 and 7 for a set of record sheets which can be used to record the task-centred work). With proper safeguards, this record can provide shared learning. The focus of these records is the process and outcome for the service users and carers, but practitioners and students can reflect on these accounts to enhance their own learning, too. The task-centred record also provides agencies with systematically collected information.

Evidence of learning must be linked to evidence that the learning has had an impact on practice. In other words, what is different as a result of the learning? Some evidence might come as self-report in supervision sessions. The portfolio is especially valuable because it 'captures' the impact of the learning in ways which others can judge.

> The main thing I learned from this session was not to underestimate a service user's ability to identify what could work for them. I realised that my role was not to choose tasks for the client, but rather to enable the client to choose the most workable options for her. . . . Is there any correlation between the lowest score (Task C) and the way we didn't use the Task Planning and Implementation Sequence for this task, as compared to Task A [where we used TPIS and got a full self-rating score]?. . . . Note: when the TPIS *was* applied to Task C in a later session, it was more successful and indeed scored a '4' when reviewed again.
>
> (Portfolio A 2000: 4.1; 4.3; 4.2)

The portfolio facilitates a dialogue with oneself, but a dialogue which can be shared with colleagues and supervisors to ensure that the reflections are not merely self-confirming.

> The portfolio is . . . an invitation to a dialogue. It is a discussion which the learner has with him- or herself, a kind of reflective soliloquy. In common

> with a soliloquy, we all know that this dialogue with oneself, though seemingly private, is held before an audience. It is not just the content which is important, but also the quality of the dialogue as a dialogue.
>
> (Doel *et al.* 2002: 50).

Prompts such as those illustrated in Box 5.1 encourage appropriately critical reflections on practice. The question 'What have you learned about your own practice from this stage in the task-centred model? triggers the following observation:

> In the past [before learning about task-centred work], to save time, I would have taken him [the service user] for his photograph. This way the onus is on Dave and it will be interesting to see if he will actually make the effort and go to [Townville] for the photograph.
>
> (Portfolio E 2000: 2.3)

Another worker reflects on her learning about the service user's capabilities:

> I have learned through the task-centred work that Sharon enjoys thinking things through at home, writing things down, and reporting back.
>
> (Portfolio A 2000: 5.2)

In response to the portfolio question, 'What similarities and what differences are there between your task-centred work and your other work?':

> More detailed analysis of the mandate for work, i.e *who is the client?*
> Explaining the method of work to be undertaken.
> Involving identified family members in the work.
> Actually undertaking direct work with the family, as opposed to assessment.
>
> (Portfolio D 2002: 2.1)

A practitioner reflects on the way her understanding of 'partnership' has changed:

> I have always attempted in my practice to work in partnership with service users, however [until] practising the task-centred approach I feel I hadn't fully took the meaning 'partnership' on board . . . I feel to some degree that [in my previous practice] I have identified problems for service users.
>
> (Portfolio D 2002: 2.3)

The emotional dimension to learning is present throughout the experience, even when risks have been successfully taken. The practitioner below demonstrates her learning that one sequence of task-centred work *can* make a difference, but that the learning will need reinforcement, sometimes by continuing work with the practitioner, sometimes by people taking on this method themselves or with or without the help of other people in their lives.

> At the start of the [final] evaluation process I made the assumption that Kelly would be very pleased with her completion of the goal. It did not occur to me that she would continue to doubt her ability. As the result of this assumption I had to think on my feet and enable Kelly to recognise her strengths and the achievements she had made while acknowledging that her thoughts were also valid. This provided me with a valuable lesson in the danger of making assumptions and [the value of] joint evaluations with service users.
>
> (Portfolio B 2002: 5.1)

Further evidence of learning comes from a greater awareness of the impact which other professional contacts have on the situation. Effective task-centred practice should make sure that other workers who are involved with the service users and carers are kept informed about the nature of the task-centred agreement, and where appropriate are directly involved in it. However, where people are locked into previous 'diagnoses', these may need unblocking in order for people to take a fresh look at their situation:

> As a result of this [task-centred] experience I will take into account previous professional contacts that service users have experienced and will take into account that their own statement of problems may have been heavily influenced by other professionals' diagnosis of problems in the past.
>
> (Portfolio F 2003: 5.1)

Evidence of learning may not become manifest until some time later, when certain connections and associations are made which help the learning make practical sense. It may, therefore, take some time for this penny to drop (see Activity 5.5).

ACTIVITY 5.5: LEARNER

Is it making a difference? Possible indicators

- How would you know whether your learning about task-centred practice is making a difference for the people you are working with? Make a note of some specific indicators that you and they could use to demonstrate the impact of this learning.
- How would you know whether your learning about task-centred practice is making a difference to your professional practice? Again, give some specific indicators which you and others could use.

There is an example answer in the Appendix.

Generalising and transferring the learning

Our understanding of the longer-term impact of new learning is largely unresearched, not just in task-centred practice but in other areas of professional learning (Rushton and Martyn 1990; Marsh and Tresiliotis 1996; Cree and Macaulay 2000). The effort to sustain a change to task-centred work should not be underestimated, especially when the stimulus of workshops, tutor interest and portfolio reflections are no longer available. As with any new learning, repeated practice is necessary for task-centred methods to become established.

It is difficult to know how many practitioners continue to use the method systematically beyond the early flower of enthusiasm, though it is common to see indications of workers beginning to generalise from the specific task-centred experience and to transfer their learning to 'everyday work':

> I have learned many very practical ideas [from the task-centred course] that I can use in everyday work. . . . This includes asking people to reflect back to

> me what they understand that I have asked them; not offering solutions too soon, to avoid suggesting what people have already tried; using the 'continuum of achievability' to assess the degree of control or chance of change; shifting the focus of problems from the person to the inter-relationship of behaviours; and re-framing actions to a positive paradigm, using the strengths model. For example, in a recent review of the care package of a young man with learning difficulties, 'Sam', it was noted that the support worker failed to meet him in a pre-arranged place. Sam had got the bus home and found the worker waiting there for him. Instead of focusing on the failure of the support worker, I drew everyone's attention to the fact that Sam had coped extremely well with an unexpected problem; he had got the bus independently, something he has not previously done. I successfully used this opportunity to highlight Sam's strengths and build on these.
>
> (Portfolio J 2002: 2.3)

> I have started . . . taking service users' work files into sessions and explaining the sections where information is kept, and why I need to keep such information. Although often surprised by this, I have experienced several different responses, from total disinterest *[sic]* to a very keen interest in reading what has been written down.
>
> (Portfolio F 2003: 5.3)

Workers also note secondary gains with the people they work with, i.e. improvements which were not the focus of the task-centred work but have nevertheless been prompted by it.

> I feel there were other benefits the family had gained during the task-centred work. The family were now communicating more and expressing feelings that they hadn't expressed previously . . . Diana felt she had learnt new ways of problem solving, and that she would use these new skills when faced with other problems.
>
> (Portfolio D 2002: 5.1; 5.2)

ACTIVITY 5.6: MANAGER

What is a learning organisation?

Sandra is a senior manager in a social care organisation. She is aware of the notion of a 'learning organisation' but is unclear what a learning organisation actually looks like and how to achieve it.

- How would you describe 'a learning organisation' to Sandra, and what would indicate that her agency was on the way to becoming one?
- In what ways could task-centred practice help Sandra to develop and implement a strategy to move her organisation towards becoming a learning organisation?

Group learning

Much of the value of the programme we outlined in Chapter 4 comes from the opportunity for participants to learn from each other. Our experience of workshops which bring people together from different specialisms and with different degrees of experience (with and without professional qualifications) has been universally positive. Many staff in social care and social work have noted that most training is 'instrumental' and focuses on statutory duties and new policy initiatives. The task-centred workshops are often the only ones where they can learn together with colleagues from different specialisms and sectors, and this is valued.

The partnerships of paired workers is a further encouragement to learning. Checking out queries and understandings with the partner, co-working with service users and carers, being a critical friend to each other when writing the portfolio, and sharing supervision, all of these provide greater support for learners. There is also an element of positive peer pressure between workshops; the commitment to presenting progress on work at the next set of workshops is a spur to getting started.

Groups are more likely to generate a wider range of options and perspectives than an individual, and to challenge each others' beliefs and assumptions. The kind of self-affirmation which can take place when practice is 'private' and unexposed is less likely when learning in groups. Group supervision or consultation can help people to develop yardsticks of good practice and fine tune their judgements. Caspi and Reid (2002: 288) note, in respect of task-centred supervision with students and staff, that 'a supervisee [learner] may continually give low ratings to their task performance yet be learning rapidly. Another may rate their task implementation highly and not be accurate or be advancing their learning'. Feedback from a group of peers can have a greater impact than from tutors or supervisors in shaping self-assessments. Involving service users and carers in these group experiences would expand the range of perspectives even further.

KEY POINTS

- ☐ It is important to start where the learner is.
- ☐ If it does not *feel* different, then it is not different; some 'unlearning' is often necessary and the process can at first feel deskilling.
- ☐ Learning is an emotional as well as a cognitive activity and it involves risk and challenge; this involves risk-taking by all involved.
- ☐ The opportunity to reflect on practice feeds back into the learning, which in turn influences the subsequent practice.
- ☐ Hindsight can be used positively to encourage alternatives and new practices for the future.
- ☐ Repeated practice and much support is necessary for new learning to become established practice, and this can be enhanced by group learning.

KEY READING

Atkins, J. (2002) 'The emotional dimension of learning' *Learning in Health and Social Care* **1**(1): 61–62

Jo Atkins usefully explores the emotional aspects of learning.

Doel, M., Sawdon, C. and Morrison, D. (2002) *Learning, Practice and Assessment: Signposting the Portfolio* London: Jessica Kingsley

This presents a holistic model which encompasses and integrates the processes of learning, practice and assessment. The discussion about the use of portfolios and 'dialogues with oneself' is helpful.

CHAPTER 6

DO

OBJECTIVES

By the end of this chapter you should:

- Have an understanding of task-centred practice in context
- Know how to build tangible partnerships built on shared knowledge
- Be able to explore problems as a basis for further work
- Work collectively towards agreed goals
- Plan and implement tasks collaboratively.

CONTEXT

Task-centred practice is relatively easily isolated in the pages of a book, but it is rather more complex to take the words off the page and to *do*. This complexity arises from the many contextual factors which have an impact on task-centred working.

Let us consider three broad contexts in turn: first, the context for the service user and carer; second, the practitioner context; and third, the agency context.

Service user and carer context

When people arrive at the doors of an agency, or when the agency arrives at their door, there is seldom a clean sheet. Past experiences of one another and current assumptions colour the encounter. The emotional context, crisis or chronic, is often especially strong.

Shame, anger, confusion and frustration are not uncommon and it is usually important for these feelings to be expressed. These contextual factors must be considered and acknowledged, including people's current explanation of their situation. These different 'worldviews' are critical (see Box 6.1).

BOX 6.1: CONTEXTS FOR PRACTICE

Example of the service user context

Sharon used to work as a teacher before having her children and was worried that we would think she should know how to manage her child's behaviour and shouldn't be experiencing difficulties. This gave an opportunity to discuss values and reassure Sharon she wasn't being judged. In fact, we admired her strength in being able to ask for help.

(Portfolio A 2000: 2.1)

Example of the practitioner context

[As the mental health support worker, I] was just given the brief to monitor the stability of John's mental health, due to his recent non-compliance with medication . . . John did not acknowledge that any problems he had were due to his illness, and refused to see his psychiatrist.

(Portfolio K 2002: 2.1)

Example of the agency context

Unfortunately the time limit [for achieving the goal] wasn't mutually agreed as I am also operating within the parameters of the existing structure of the Centre for Pre-5 Year Old's, and also the time restrictions regarding caseload and working on a job-share basis . . . it remains to be seen what kind of effect an imposed time limit will have on this piece of work.

(Portfolio A 2000: 3.2)

Some service users and carers know the agency well and some may even be residents in the agency. One task-centred practitioner describes a resident, Roger, as

> a 30-yr old man with learning disabilities. He has autism and cerebral palsy and requires the use of a wheelchair. Roger is non-verbal; however, the changing pitch of his voice and vocal expressions can be identified by staff and enable them to meet or respond to his needs. . . . Prioritising Roger's problems was achieved by accessing a knowledge base accumulated by support staff over a three year period.
>
> (Portfolio I 2003: 2.1; 2.3)

Roger may have been non-verbal, but he was vocal and his carers' long-standing personal knowledge of him was essential for them to be able to use the task-centred model in their work with him.

Task-centred practice encourages an understanding of people in their wider context, including the social policies which have an impact on their personal situations. Their experience of disadvantage and discrimination, and the differences in 'social location' between users, carers and practitioners will all have an impact on this first and subsequent encounters. The social supports (or lack of them) in the wider family and community are also crucial to this context. Mobilising possible supports is an important strategy, especially to sustain future efforts and to maintain the momentum after the work has been completed. The relative 'size and weight' of this support will help to determine the ambition or modesty of the overall goal.

Practitioner context

There are many contextual factors for practitioners. The obvious ones concern time, space and support to learn and practise the model. However, we need more research to understand how some practitioners are able to foster task-centred practice despite the pressure of work.

As the example in Box 6.1 demonstrates, workers are subject to pressures from other practitioners. The collaboration of inter-professional working can cross a line into collusion. In this case, peer pressure pushed the worker to ensure that John took his medication. The worker felt compelled to challenge John's own definition of himself as a person with a problem, and to support (or collude?) with the professional view of John as a person with an illness. However, the spirit of task-centred practice entails more careful listening to John's self-definition. Once the model had been explained to John, he understood this, too.

These differences are sometimes described as 'narratives' (Weingarten 1998). A practitioner is part of a wider professional community, in which there are also many different values, perspectives and narratives. Service users and carers will vary in the degree to which they differentiate between the various professionals who might play a part in their lives, now or in the past, and the task-centred practitioner needs to be mindful of this.

> Kelly and Tina told me of their lesbian relationship on our first meeting . . . Kelly told a story of several years ago when after a lengthy period [in a mental hospital] the consultant told her that the reason for her mental illhealth was her sexuality!
>
> (Portfolio B 2002: 6)

Another significant part of this context is the view held by the practitioner of what task-centred practice is. Some of the misconceptions about task-centred work are illustrated in Box 6.2, which indicates how a 'stick-on' task-centred approach is doomed from the start and undermines the reputation of the model. If we are to build a database comparable to Reid's (2000) Task Planner, we need to be confident that what is labelled 'task-centred' *is* task-centred.

BOX 6.2: WHAT 'TASK-CENTRED' IS *NOT*

The following extract is taken from a PQ1* social work portfolio:

> After sharing my concerns with my manager, it was agreed that I should adopt a 'task-centred approach' with this family to encourage them to improve their health, hygiene and overall environment. [The portfolio our own inverted commas].

From the same portfolio:

> Initially I was able to engage with the family and set up a programme of work, which set tasks for them to complete. The aim was for the tasks to be time limited and be completed in manageable chunks in order that they were not overwhelmed by their situation and to enable the family to feel that they were achieving, and improve their self-esteem.

Later, from the same portfolio:

> From the outset, there were difficulties in the tasks being completed, little improvement was noted and there were always excuses for work not being done.

And later:

> I became very aware of my own value base and questioned myself as to whether I was being too hard on this family and that their living arrangements were based upon my own experiences.

Note: *PQ1 is the first stage of all qualified social workers' continuing professional development in the UK. This example is, therefore, taken from a general portfolio, not a task-centred one. See Activity 6.1.

ACTIVITY 6.1: LEARNER

What is *not* task-centred practice and why?

- Why is the example in Box 6.2 *not* an example of task-centred work? Make a note of your reasons, including what you think is missing from this example and what it would need to turn it into an example of task-centred practice.
- Return to this question after you have completed reading this chapter and the next (Review). Are there any further elements which you would add to your list?

Agency context

As we noted in the Introduction to this book, in many respects, task-centred practice has come of age. It is a method with partnership at its heart, built on a substantial evidence base and accountable to others. Yet the challenges to successful task-centred practice in agencies are considerable.

An effort to hold professionals to better account, by increasing regulation at the practitioner level, is having effects which sometimes appear perverse from the point of view of encouraging good practice; for example, estimates that social workers spend only one hour in eight in direct contact with service users and carers. Task-centred practice does, of course, require practitioners to *do*. Although it takes account of context, it is essentially a face-to-face contact model of professional practice. Ironically, it holds professionals to account far more effectively than external regulation ever can, it provides untold detail and information for those agencies which choose to collate it, and it is does this efficiently because the paperwork is completed there and then, in-session (see Chapter 7). In the search for evidence-based practice, we are in danger of neglecting what lies under our noses. Perhaps it is too much to expect government ministers and officials to read this book!

There is no doubt that the current agency context is not hospitable to the systematic development and use of a practice method such as task-centred work. Overwhelmed by regulation and public expectation, tearing itself apart with the perpetual revolution of reorganisation and restructuring, and barely out of the ark in terms of new technology, this is not promising territory. Agencies and their workers are drowning in new initiatives and vast assessment documents, all designed to be 'needs-led' and 'user-friendly', yet with little of the elegance or accessibility of the task-centred documentation and methodology. Though the format of the task-centred recording is relatively 'light touch', the extra energy needed to gear it to the assessment documentation devised by central authorities can be the last straw (Department of Health 2000, 2002).

If we can turn this corner, task-centred practice has enormous potential. As we have noted, it makes practice accountable to the people who use it, to the agency and to central authorities. At a time when only one in twenty of low-skilled employees is offered training, compared to one in four of those with degrees (*Guardian Education*, 9 March 2004), it provides a method which has been learned and used by many unqualified, as well as qualified, staff.

Agencies may have a perception of task-centred practice as something that can only be used with relatively 'easy' cases, and therefore not see its mainstream potential. While it is true that there are limits to the possibilities of task-centred practice (as there are with any practice method), task-centred principles are always applicable. The experience of several hundred practitioners on various task-centred training courses (see Chapter 4) has shown its flexibility in very difficult and varied situations (see Activity 6.2).

ACTIVITY 6.2: MANAGER

Promoting task-centred practice as the primary method of choice

You have just been appointed operational manager for field services in your agency. You believe that the evidence base for task-centred practice is strong and you wish to promote its use as the primary method of choice in your agency.

- What strengths does your agency have which would support a strategy to develop and support task-centred practice?
- What weaknesses do you see which could fail to support or even undermine such a strategy?
- What opportunities are there to take the strategy forward?
- What might threaten the strategy, from both inside and outside the agency?

PARTNERSHIP, AUTHORITY, POWER AND OPPRESSION

> John said, 'I feel like I am gaining control of my situation before we have even started.'
>
> (Portfolio K 2002: 3)

A tangible partnership built on shared knowledge

'Partnership' is an omnipresent term in the literature and the legislation, but through the task-centred portfolios we have tangible evidence of what it means in practice. For example, a worker who uses flipcharts as part of her general work, comments on the differences she found using a flipchart in the task-centred model:

> I have found [using the flipchart] has been very different in the task-centred process, as there has been no need to record anything separately afterwards. All the information on the flip sheets has been explanation enough. This also had the advantage of Sharon always being able to see what was written and provided opportunity for her to request I change it if I recorded anything inaccurately. . . . If we are advocating working in partnership, then surely the recording should be done together . . . This is 'the real thing', a joint process between practitioner and client, that should stand on its own merit, and not merely be used as a tool to write up the 'real' session afterwards.
>
> (Portfolio A 2000: 5.3)

The need to work closely together in task-centred practice can sometimes even be mirrored in the physical positions adopted during a session. For example, one worker noted that 'we were both sat on the floor [to make notes] which worked well, as it gave a feeling of equality' (Portfolio K 2002: 2.2). We will consider how to record the work and the use of flipcharts in Chapter 7.

Partnership is built on shared knowledge and information. A key aspect of this is the involvement of service users and carers in knowledge of the task-centred method itself, and the way in which it works. People will have different degrees of interest and ability, but everyone is encouraged to learn as much as they want or can about how and why task-centred practice works. Information is, indeed, power.

> He seemed to have a very good understanding of the principles of the [task-centred] practice and I found that on a number of occasions John was finishing my sentences for me while I was explaining the process.
>
> (Portfolio K 2002: 2.2)

Contrasting the new experience of joint recording with a family when using the task-centred method, another practitioner noted that usually 'only if the family made a request to see their file would they normally read what is written about them' (Portfolio D 2002: 5.3). Although the Access to Personal Files Act was passed in 1987, allowing service users to see their records, 'very few people actually take up on this opportunity' and when they do, it is often 'in retrospect in order to find out specific pieces of information' (Portfolio F 2003: 5.3).

An equal partnership?

Some writers suggest that the differences in power between workers, users and carers can never allow a true partnership, even that task-centred practice 'supports managerialist objectives' (Dominelli 1996: 156). Of course, there are real constraints on partnership and none ever achieves absolute 'equality', since each party to a partnership brings different qualities and different powers. However, the power profile is far more complex than a simple set of scales, and this is true of all social work encounters. In some cases the constraints are clear, such as legally mandated work, but even then there are other power dynamics at play; for example, a newly qualified, black female social worker might disagree that the legal mandate gives her *all* the power in the face of an aggressive, white male offender.

The differences and the distances are likely to be seen at their starkest at the beginning of the encounter. Indeed, task-centred practitioners ensure that issues of power and oppression are open and explicit, part of the weave of the work. The task-centred process aims to move *towards* partnership; the speed and degree of success will vary enormously from one situation to another.

> My work with Wayne was legally mandated and his initial compliance with our work probably reflected his fear of the consequences should he not comply. By the end of our work, I believe that Wayne and I experienced a true sense of working in partnership.
>
> (Portfolio F 2003: 5)

This same practitioner reflected on the great differences between herself and the service user:

> On meeting for the first time, Wayne and I could identify little common ground. Wayne is a mixed race male teenager with drug misuse problems and a significant criminal record. I am a white, middle aged, female social worker who has statutory responsibility for enforcing an order made by the courts. In terms of the outcome, I am not sure whether this would have been affected to any great extent had I been a black, male worker who had previously overcome drug or offending issues. It seems that despite our differences, Wayne and I did engage and work in partnership to achieve significant progress in addressing his problems.
>
> (Portfolio F 2003: 6)

Task-centred work can bring people together to transcend the differences in their biographies. Practitioners entering into the world of other people cannot and should not 'live' those worlds, but they can and should be sensitive to them, including for example task-centred terminology; one practitioner referred to tasks as 'jobs' and others used people's colloquialisms to record the work together.

Part of the inequality in the partnership is the worker's authority, and it is crucial that there is no attempt to deny or belittle this difference. Indeed, this authority is often essential to the success of the work; to deny or suppress it is not just dishonest, but a wasted opportunity. The work depends on harnessing this authority, both 'inside' the task-centred encounter and 'outside', when demands are made of other practitioners, agencies and institutions (see Activity 6.3).

> If I hadn't been using the task-centred model, I might have moved the work at Sharon's fast pace, which may have removed the opportunity for her to explore some of the problems and ultimately address them.
>
> (Portfolio A 2000: 2.2)

> Wayne was enabled to decide which tasks he could complete himself and which he would like me to do. Our partnership meant that he took on what he felt able to cope with and I did the rest. Wayne liked the idea of a partnership in which I was also accountable for the tasks that I had to complete. He said that he had previously been let down by workers not carrying out what they had agreed to do.
>
> (Portfolio F 2003: 6)

ACTIVITY 6.3: SERVICE USER AND CARER

What is partnership?

'Partnership' is a term often used in social work and other areas of health and social care.

- What is your idea of a partnership?
- What would show that you and your worker were working in partnership?
- How do you think task-centred practice can help to build the partnership?

Ultimately, task-centred practice is about making choices, with an honest recognition of the constraints on these choices. Some elements are not negotiable, but the work allows other choices to be formulated and other decisions to be taken. The process of the work itself will present many opportunities for people to make choices, and even those which seem relatively trivial can be significant, such as respecting a choice *not* to do something.

> Our second session focused upon returning to the headlines and detailing each problem. As in our initial session, Wayne chose not to write. Again this was due to Wayne's lack of confidence in his ability to write without making mistakes. (Despite my coaxing, Wayne never felt able to write during any of our work) . . .

> . . . Wayne commented that it was unusual for a worker to offer him this type of information, in his previous community supervision programmes he felt that he was told 'what' to do rather than 'why'.
>
> (Portfolio F 2003: 5.3; 2.2)

Task-centred work makes the worker engage with the service user and carer's moral world, with an increased understanding of how that world is explained. More than just respecting that world, it means entering it and according it status and power. We do not know how John (below) felt when, at his own insistence, his worker crossed out the word 'illness' and substituted it for 'problem', but we can guess that it was strongly affirming and that it moved the partnership one step nearer to that elusive notion of 'equalness'.

> John asked me to change the odd word as he did not like the image it gave, for example, I *had to* change the word illness to problem.
>
> (Portfolio K 2002: 2.2 – our emphasis)

There is perhaps nothing more empowering than experiencing someone else having confidence in you. One of the many positive commitments which practitioners give through their task-centred practice is 'the message, "*I know you can begin to see a way out of this difficulty and I have confidence you can carry this out*"' (Portfolio A 2000: 1.3). This commitment is not given *carte blanche,* but after a careful analysis of just what is and what is not possible and desirable, and within what timescale; to do anything else would be irresponsible, but once this agreement has been made, on the basis of shared knowledge and understanding, it can prove powerful and empowering (see Activity 6.4).

ACTIVITY 6.4: SUPERVISOR

Ensuring participation: the role of task-centred practice

The following quotation from a foster carer is taken from a social worker's dissertation on a research project which explored the role of foster carers in young people leaving care:

> Mrs Lee said she felt she had been quite involved in planning for some of the young people she had fostered, but marginalised in the planning for others. *She felt it depended on the social worker if they included her or not*, and that there was also a problem with the shortage of social workers as there was a lack of continuity and support for the young person in transition. [our emphasis]

The quotation demonstrates that social workers have considerable power and authority. In the light of this:

- How would you ensure that it didn't '*depend on the social worker if they included her or not*'?
- What role could task-centred practice play in preventing this?

PROBLEMS

'People are forced to solve problems but no-one is ever forced to look for opportunities. However, every-one is *free* to look for opportunities – if they so wish' (Bono 2000: 108, discussing 'yellow hat' thinking).

The first stage of task-centred practice is exploring problems. This stage consists of a general scan of the current problems in the person's life and an attempt to prioritise these by discussing them in detail. Practitioners can also note any additional problems which the person might not have identified. A maximum of three problems (and usually just one or two) is selected for work. See Chapter 2 for more details.

Is history important?

Exploring problems with people is not a neutral activity. All problems have a context which is often emotion laden and history bound.

> Evelyn had experienced money problems for many years. When we explored this with her, she dated the problem back to when both her parents had died quite suddenly, and within a few months of each other, eight years previously. They had clearly been her main means of support both with her children and in financial matters and she felt that since this time she had found it difficult to prioritise and use her money effectively.
>
> (Portfolio G 2000: 3.2)

One of the fundamental dilemmas facing the practitioner is how far to delve into the history of a problem. In Evelyn's case above, how far should we explore the events of eight years ago and to what depth should we enquire about the feelings evoked by the loss of her parents? Quite simply, the guiding principle for task-centred work is the focus on the here-and-now.

The dilemma for the task-centred practitioner is that the service user or carer may *want* to focus on the past, or has learned to do this. Of course, a person's past should not be dismissed, and their desire to put current problems into context should be respected. The task-centred practitioner can gently focus questions around the person's *problem-solving history*, since past attempts to solve current problems are very relevant. In these circumstances the worker can explain that, though an understanding of the past can be illuminating, a focus on the present will be necessary if the problem is to be solved, or at least reduced, and that it will be unhelpful to dig back and deep for an elusive 'root cause'.

One line of practice wisdom suggests that problems will reoccur if the root cause remains; indeed, this horticultural metaphor has a powerful hold, with images of problems resprouting like Russian vine if not thoroughly excised. Certainly, there are examples of recurring problems, but it is by no means clear that this is due to a failure to tackle some deeper cause. There are many other possible explanations, including the fact that lives are not lived problem free, deep or otherwise, and that some people have more difficulty than others in learning and using problem-solving techniques.

More significant than the histories are the meanings and associations which people attribute to their problems. It is this ecological approach to problems rather than an historical one which is most effective and the main guide for task-centred practice. This does not mean that historical insights cannot benefit present problem-solving, but the focus remains on the latter, not the former.

> Evelyn was able to recognise that she was treating Carl, her eldest child, in the same way her parents had with her, i.e. he was relying on her to pay off debts [despite the fact that Carl was claiming his own benefit].
>
> (Portfolio G 2000: 3.2)

Focusing on the here-and-now can often be a considerable relief to people. There may be long-standing problems which will not be solved by the current work, but service users and carers may not wish to work on them, or to work only on parts of them. The root and branch practice wisdom is countered by the evidence from task-centred and solution-focused methods, which indicate that problem separation and discrimination is possible, even desirable. If the problem is identified as 'the copper beech tree', because its shade chokes off the plants beneath, the solution may not be to uproot the whole tree, but to cut back some of the branches. Over time they will grow again, but once I know how to cut them back, I can do so again.

> Wayne's mother, Sue, has told me that Wayne has problems with self harming/mutilation and soiling problems which started when he went into custody as a direct result of bullying that he experienced while in the Young Offenders Institution. Wayne is deeply embarrassed about both issues and does not wish to discuss or address either problem at present.
>
> (Portfolio F 2003: 2.2)

How deep should we dig? There is no reason to doubt the line of causality which Wayne's mother has drawn, but the 'problem' would then become the regime in a Young Offenders Institution – an important target for change, but probably unrealistic for Wayne and his worker, especially if we are concerned to respect Wayne's wishes. Moreover, changes in past 'causes' of present problems do not necessarily help with current problems; would changes at the Young Offenders Institution make any difference now to Wayne's current problems?

Selecting the problem

> [Exploring all the different problems and writing them down] helped us to see that on the one hand each headline was a problem in its own right, but on the other hand they had components that affected each other. For example, his drug use and poor temper control made him more likely to offend.
>
> (Portfolio F 2003: 2.2)

At one level, the ability to understand the complex relationship between different problems while also discriminating between them, is crucial to effective task-centred practice. Selecting a problem which is key to the current difficulties, yet is amenable to change within a restricted time period, is a complex matter. Even so, examples of practitioners' task-centred work indicates effective use of the model with people with a wide range of abilities and circumstances, from people whose intellectual grasp of the model is immediate, to others whose cognition is severely limited and, in one instance, where communication depends on vocalisation rather than verbalisation.

The therapeutic value of one person's concern for another is well documented (Egan 1986) and there is no doubt that the attention and regard which is the gift of the task-centred practitioner, seems capable of transcending difficulties in cognition. Indeed, the strength of the partnership seems no weaker in cases where it is only the worker who is able to grasp the task-centred processes than in those situations where there is a 'cognitive partnership' as well. The model has to be highly adapted in different circumstances, but central to its strength and effectiveness, is the worker's concern for the people they work with. This can lead to people being very honest with themselves:

> I *am* intelligent, it's just the way I look.
>
> (Portfolio K 2002: 2.2)

As we explained in Chapter 2, the worker's concern is made manifest in the detailed exploration of each of the current problem areas in the person's life. The worker conducts this dialogue without enforced judgement and without solutions and strategies. It is a structured narrative which, when done well, does not feel structured, and one in which people are encouraged to draw a picture (sometimes literally) of their current life problems; sketching at first, then more detail, with an increasing understanding of the connections (see Boxes 6.3 and 6.4 and Activity 6.5). From this process, one problem is selected for detailed work (or occasionally two or three), on the basis that the person feels motivated to work on this problem, that it is reasonably specific, that it is capable of some degree of resolution, and that it is considered desirable by all involved to work on this problem. Workers' expertise is focused not on selecting the problem for the person, but on helping to cast light on which of the problems may be key to others. This is not necessarily the biggest, most important or obvious problem.

BOX 6.3: EXAMPLE OF EXPLORING PROBLEMS: JOHN

Date of this session: 18 October

Persons involved: John (service user), Gwen (worker)

Problem chosen to work on (the selected problem):
'I used to have a right active, outgoing life; I can't get used to this now.'

Details of this problem:

What? John finds it very difficult to socialise and experience new activities due to a lack of confidence and the knowledge that he hasn't done so for a number of years.

Who? John is the only individual involved in this problem. John gets very frustrated, as he tends to remember his life before his illness, when he was very active and outgoing.

When? John is affected daily by his problem as he feels unable to experience new activities and environments. John became withdrawn and lacked confidence around the time of his first psychotic episode. John lost his business, a driving school, and his family due to his illness, and as a result became quite withdrawn and lacking confidence. Gradually over time John has isolated himself.

Where? John now only feels comfortable going to the betting shop and the local market. He feels unable to go anywhere else.

Why? John feels it was the stress of the responsibilities he had in the past, owning his own driving school, which made him become unwell and withdraw from society. John now feels that he needs new social stimulation in order to keep his mind active. John has very little insight into his illness and prefers to classify it as a problem rather than an illness, which he feels is only kept at bay if his mind is kept active and stimulated. At present, John keeps his mind active by doing mathematics exercises at home and going to the bookies to study the form.

How? John feels that by experiencing new activities his mind will be kept active and stimulated, which will contribute to subduing his 'problem'. John hopes that he may meet some new acquaintance and be able to have a stimulating conversation.

Other problems included in the problem scan, but not being worked on at present:
None at present.

(Portfolio K 2002: 2.3)

BOX 6.4: EXAMPLE OF EXPLORING PROBLEMS: WAYNE

Date of this session: 25 November

Persons involved: Wayne (service user), Barbara (worker)

Problem chosen to work on (the selected problem):
Violence and aggression.

Details of this problem:

What? Wayne easily loses his temper, threatens violence and on occasions has carried out threats by hitting people.

Who? Wayne has threatened violence towards his mother. He has been violent towards his siblings, neighbours, friends and strangers.

When? Over the last three years, consistently. At different times of day or night.

Where? In the family home and outside the home.

Why? Wayne often feels angry about his circumstances and loses his temper. His misuse of heroin makes him more likely to lose his temper when he is withdrawing. Wayne has become used to responding aggressively and does not have the alternative skills to manage his behaviour.

How? Wayne shouts in people's faces, bangs doors, hits, punches, kicks etc.

Other problems included in the problem scan, but not being worked on at present: Insomnia.

(Portfolio F 2003: 2.3)

> She saw this [selected problem] as one that affected many areas of her life, including her ability to provide adequately for her children [who had been accommodated] and her own mental health.
>
> (Portfolio G 2000: 2.3)

A factor which can also help the person in their selection is the consequence of not working on a particular problem:

Evelyn's children would not be returned to her until she moved to a more suitable property. She therefore needed to pay off her arrears and would need to budget and prioritise her money towards this end.

(Portfolio G 2000: 2.3)

ACTIVITY 6.5: PRACTITIONER

Being specific

We know that being *specific* increases the chances of success in resolving a problem. Choose one of the two examples of a selected problem (Boxes 6.3 and 6.4) and rewrite it so that it is more specific. Use your imagination to create additional information as appropriate.

There is an example answer in the Appendix.

Additional problems

The 'inadequate housing' identified by the workers as an additional problem was entirely consistent with Evelyn's problem that her rent arrears meant that she was unable to find the better housing she desired. This was a situation she had lived with and come to accept – she felt powerless to change it and had not thought to list it as a problem as it seemed to her something she could do nothing about.

(Portfolio G 2000: 2.2)

Social workers see themselves as helpers, but they are often involved with people who find the help is being imposed on them. Any method of practice must be capable of accommodating the dual role of social work, as care and control. For this reason, workers need to include the notion of 'additional problems' in their explanation of how task-centred practice works. When exploring problems together, workers also have the right and responsibility to lay their concerns on the table. It is usually best to do this *after* the service user or carer, so that the problem areas which the worker has identified do not set the agenda and because it is becomes possible to reframe these problems into the service user's language and worldview at this later stage. However, people need to know beforehand that the worker may present additional identified problems.

The process of reframing problems is significant in developing the alliance between workers, users and carers. The worker might have 'poor care of the children' as the reason for their intervention and this may not be articulated as a problem by the service user during the exploration stage, but it is highly likely that related problems will have been. One service user saw 'housework, money and leaving the kids with Alan' as problems. In fact, these reflected quite accurately the workers' concerns, though they needed to reframe their own concerns in order to see this.

It seemed that practical issues rather than childcare and the children's welfare took precedence for her. However, we were in agreement that these were problem areas, and on further exploration I felt that Evelyn had in fact simplified many of the workers' concerns very well:

- 'Housework' – workers were concerned about the poor housing conditions, safety within the home, lack of hygiene, poor diet.
- 'Money' – workers were concerned that Evelyn was unable to provide basic care such as heating, food, clothes, bedding.
- 'Leaving the kids with Alan' – workers were concerned about the lack of adult supervision and leaving the children with inappropriate adults.

(Portfolio G 2000: 2.2)

Giving people the time and space to express the problems in the way they see them is important because a joint interrogation of the facts is more likely to enhance motivation for future work than a presentation of the facts as the worker sees them; and, far from the opportunity for manipulation which some practitioners fear, it can be a challenging process for all involved. Rather than putting the service user into a position of defending their corner, the problem exploration phase encourages engagement, and with that engagement comes the likelihood of more openness by everyone involved.

> Wayne had chosen the three key problem areas in his life that were putting him at risk of custody [and he] was able to recognise that all three problems were interlinked, the most influential feature being the 'drug misuse'. . . . Despite being labelled as a 'persistent' young offender, having his liberty removed and being subject to strict community supervision, I was surprised and impressed by Wayne's ability to separate his behaviour from his personal identity. Wayne stated in our problem detailing session that he is a strong and mainly 'good person' who wants to change his way of behaving. . . . [Wayne] has been parented by Sue, a black woman, with a strong cultural identity who both confronts and challenges structures in society which label people. It appears that she has given constant reassurance to Wayne of his positive qualities and ability to succeed despite his substantial problems in life.
>
> (Portfolio F 2003: 2.3)

As the following quote indicates, most people are wise to probable 'additional problems':

> Despite the fact that Wayne suggested this [the heroin problem] himself in the problem scan, I suspect that he was offering the suggestion to address the drug misuse as a way of appearing to be complying with the legal mandate and meeting my expectations as his supervising officer.
>
> (Portfolio F 2003: 5.1)

Avoiding giving solutions

Well-intentioned practitioners can sometimes find it difficult to rein in their desire to provide a solution. We know what worked for someone else and, as soon as the person begins to describe a particular problem, our mental card index of possible solutions is flipping wildly. While this is happening we are not listening to the person exploring their problem, and when we deliver the solution ('I think you should try . . .?'; 'Why don't you consider . . .?') it has the opposite effect to that desired. The service user's lack of enthusiasm is then interpreted as negativism, and frequently there is a deepening gulf as the worker presses the case for the solution against the service user's hardening opposition. Quite simply, the worker has not allowed the solution to be the user or carer's *own* solution.

Moreover, moving sharply between exploring the details of problems and searching for goals and solutions is like trying to change gear without using the clutch. There are very different 'moods' to these two processes.

> We discussed Sharon using some anger management techniques at home but Sharon felt she had already been trying to control her temper before she sought help and it hadn't worked for her.
>
> (Portfolio A 2000: 4.1)

It is better to ask the person to consider times when they have handled the problem well, or whether there are times when it is not a problem and why that might be. Asking people to identify things they do well, or talk about times without the problem will help gently to anticipate the goal-setting phase of the work. It helps people to think about their own potential solutions, tailored to their own particular circumstances, not a quick fix from a solution toolbox.

GOALS

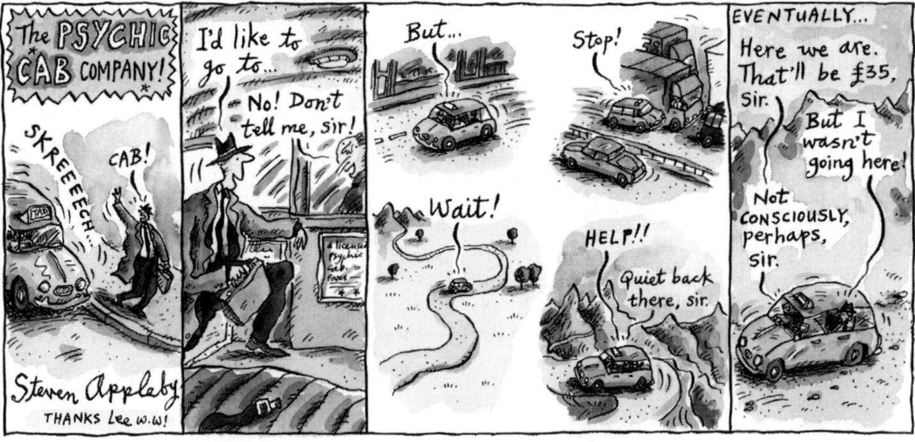

FIGURE 6.1 The Psychic Cab (courtesy of Steven Appleby)

It is through the process of negotiating a goal that people truly get a sense of their power to steer and guide the work. At all costs, the 'Psychic Cab' syndrome must be avoided (see Figure 6.1)! It is this phase which really challenges commonly held views of service users and carers as uniformly vulnerable and damaged, rather than as potential drivers to their own futures. Agreeing the goal is the greatest expression of a working partnership based on a strengths model of social work practice.

> I discussed my concerns [about whether I had unduly influenced her choice of goal] with Sharon, who felt that she truly didn't know why she kept losing her temper, so wasn't able to say for certain that achieving the selected goal would resolve the problem. However, she said that she had a strong feeling that her expectations of Tom [her son] were a large factor, and wanted to deal with

> this. She felt that it may well resolve her problem, and if it didn't, would be eliminated as a factor, indicating she needed to consider any other possible causes. We both agreed we could use the task-centred method to do this.
>
> (Portfolio A 2000: 3.2)

The dialogue between Sharon and her social worker (above) is characterised by trust and reasoning, because the worker has given a clear account of the task-centred method and has demonstrated it during the problem exploration. This has strengthened the service user's confidence, not just in the worker and the method, but also in her own capacity. It is clear that the work is harnessing Sharon's ability to reason about her situation. Commonly, we find that people who have been seen as 'difficult', 'vulnerable', 'dependent', etc. are able to make thoughtful, reasoned choices when given the opportunity and are often all too aware of the difference between a wish and a realisable want, what is possible now and what might be possible in the future. Dave, described as having mild learning difficulties and Fragile X syndrome, says, 'I want a job, I know I can't get one yet but that is what I would like' (Portfolio E 2000: 2.2).

In common with the selected problem, the chosen goal should be one which is feasible and desirable for the person to achieve within the agreed time limit, relatively specific, something they feel motivated about, and a clearly understood link between how the goal will alleviate the problem. Up to three goals may be worked on at any one time, but it is often desirable to focus on just one, especially if this is the person's first experience of task-centred work. One practitioner, working in a specialist child care team, compared her task-centred work with her previous practice and noted that, while she regularly worked with goals that were realistic, 'there have often been many more of them, thus making them less likely to be attainable' and that, in her everyday practice, 'it has been expected that the goals will somehow magically be achieved if everyone contributes to and signs the agreement' (Portfolio C 1995: 6).

Although the process of negotiating a goal has a more positive feel than exploring the problems, it can nevertheless be experienced as risky. It is at this point that people realise that their worker is taking them seriously and that the near future will require commitment, application and courage. Experiences of trust and expectations of success may be new, and feelings of fear and failure are likely to reoccur. 'Some of Evelyn's comments when negotiating the Agreement indicated how helpless she felt about her situation' (Portfolio G 2000: 3). Change means taking risks, and this applies to the worker as well as the user. Everyone will need regular reminders of the gains, not just from achieving the goal, but also from experiencing the process.

> I found negotiating an agreement quite difficult. Dave still feels that he should have someone to do the work for him, but was prepared to give the agreement a try. . . . He was actually quite elated after this session that he had made decisions and agreed the agreement.
>
> (Portfolio E 2000: 3.2)

The authors have had their own assumptions challenged about the scope of the task-centred method. For example, Roger's limited ability to communicate (he could vocalise but not verbalise) meant that his worker had to adapt the task-centred model. She gathered a list of possible goals drawn from the collective experience and knowledge of the staff team caring for Roger. These were written on flipchart paper, which she included in her portfolio:

> I wish I could wear clothes that feel good on my skin.
>
> I would like more motion activities like fairground rides, train journeys and bumper car rides.
>
> I would like to have the opportunity to experience social activities that involve my own participation – bowling, swimming, etc.
>
> I would like to distinguish between utensils needed for eating and when it is finger foods.
>
> I would like to have a say in where I go when we go on outings.
>
> I would like my meals when I am hungry and not at set times.
>
> I would like to be able to choose my own drinks when out at the pub or in the supermarket.
>
> I would like to communicate when my incontinence pad needs changing.
>
> (Portfolio I 2003: flipchart appendix)

Whether consciously or not, the use of 'I would like to' and 'I wish' rather than 'I want to' conveys the necessary sense of tentativeness to the goals, given that they are not being verbalised by Roger.

Of course, the process of moving from problem exploration to goal negotiation is not as linear as the words on a page suggest. Often, people will present their wants and aspirations while discussing their problems, and ideas for possible goals will probably already have been touched upon. However, making the agreement ensures that the act of agreeing a goal is proactive and not a default, and that a range of possibilities have been considered. It is quite common for people to have preconceived ideas about their goal (sometimes given to them by others), and the task-centred process helps everyone to step back before making the decision.

Time limits

The agreement is the crux of the task-centred work. It brings together the selected problem or problems, the chosen goal or goals, and – last but not least – the time limit for the work, which includes the expected frequency of contact. There are a number of reasons why agreeing the length of involvement is an integral aspect of the task-centred method. First, there is the effect which we all experience as we move towards a deadline (for a report, a special event, a holiday break, etc.) in which our mind concentrates on the coming event with increasing strength. A time limit is, therefore, motivating. In addition, it helps all involved to pace the work and to understand whether the rate of progress is satisfactory. Of course, most goals are not so quantifiable that the time between now and the deadline can be neatly divided up into equal sized parcels; however, it is possible to have a sense of whether the time already spent and the progress towards the goal feel proportionate. Finally, a deadline helps to prevent a sense of drift; if it has been judged reasonably accurately it can ensure that there is just the right degree of pressure to fuel the motivation. The time limit should be negotiated on the requirements of the goal (i.e. how long is it likely to take to achieve?), and this same principle determines the frequency of sessions.

It is the application of time limits and the short-term nature of much task-centred practice which has attracted critics, who see this as 'managerialist' and unsympathetic to the use of 'relationship'. It is true that short-term work has attractions for managers and agencies in terms of economy of resource; if short-term engagements can produce similar, even improved, experiences for service users and carers, it would be perverse to oppose them just because they also appeal to the drive to use resources economically. In terms of the use of relationship, we hope that by this stage in the book, readers will be in no doubt about the intensity and central importance of the relationship between the partners in task-centred work. This method builds relationships through the work together, with the relationship arising from the doing, rather than the doing arising from a relationship. We believe this mirrors what happens in our everyday lives, just as a complete stranger can feel like a lifelong friend if you happen to find yourselves mutually dependent in a short, intense crisis.

Although the time limit should be driven by the needs of the goal, the agency context which we described early in this chapter will also shape what is possible. Also, those service users and carers who are in regular and enduring contact with services may find the idea of a time limit unsettling, so it is important to emphasise that it is the specific piece of work which has the limit. In some instances, the contact will continue beyond the period of any one agreement.

> John did have a little difficulty grasping the concept of a time limit. This being because few individuals within the agency are discharged from caseloads due to the nature of our work and the severity of ill health, severe and enduring mental ill health, and as a result John has always had a worker since the onset of his illness.
>
> (Portfolio K 2002: 3.1)

Credibility is lost if time limits are easily breached and lengthened. On the other hand, flexibility is important to take account of unforeseen circumstances and other kinds of hiccup. If the goal can be achieved with an extension of time, this should be allowed; if more time is being sought because the work has gone adrift it will be better to terminate the current agreement and consider negotiating a new one which takes proper account of the changed circumstances or new knowledge (see Box 6.5). Once one particular piece of work has been completed, the worker should be prepared to consider how they would respond to a request to start another sequence:

> John enjoyed working in this way so much he has asked me if it would be possible to look at another of his problems he initially mentioned in the problem scan.
>
> (Portfolio K 2002: 5.2)

BOX 6.5: EXAMPLES OF THE AGREEMENT

Example 1

Date: 6 January
Parties to the agreement: Wayne (service user), Barbara (social worker)
The selected problem(s):
The problem I want to work on is . . . drug misuse.

The agreed goal(s):
I want to . . . be able to live my life without using heroin.
Time limit and frequency of contact:
We aim to complete this work by . . . 3 March.
We will be meeting . . . weekly; every Monday at 2 p.m.

(Portfolio F 2003: 3.1)

Example 2

Date: 30 October
Parties to the agreement: Paula (service user), Margaret (social worker)
The selected problem(s):
The problem I want to work on is . . . my bereavement due to my mum's recent death and the emotions that go with it.
The agreed goal(s):
I want to . . . have the space to come to terms with it and have a listening ear.
Time limit and frequency of contact:
We aim to complete this work by . . . after 6 weeks I will reflect and review.
We will be meeting . . . each Tuesday at 2 p.m.

(Portfolio J 2003: 3.1)

Example 3

Date: 13 November
Parties to the agreement: Roger (service user), Laura (support worker)
The selected problem(s):
The problem I want to work on is . . . I can't choose my own drinks.
The agreed goal(s):
I want to . . . choose my own drinks and drinking implement.
Time limit and frequency of contact:
We aim to complete this work by . . . 18 November.
We will be meeting . . . daily.

(Portfolio I 2003: 3.1)

Example 4

Date: 29 October
Parties to the agreement: Kelly (service user), Tina (her partner), Erica (social worker)
The selected problem(s):
The problem I want to work on is . . . my agoraphobia and inability to access public and private transport.
The agreed goal(s):
I want to . . . be able to access GP and outpatient appointments with Tina, so that I can have my medication reviewed and my mental and physical health assessed.
Time limit and frequency of contact:
We aim to complete this work by . . . 28 February.
We will be meeting . . . weekly.

(Portfolio B 2003: 3.1)

Multiple involvements

When there are a number of complex problems involving different members of a family or larger system it is necessary to consider multiple involvement in the agreement or, indeed, of creating more than one agreement. For example, in the case of the Barnes family, Mat was being hit by his older stepbrother, Daniel, who in turn was being 'wound up' by Mat, whose mother the workers felt was colluding in allowing Daniel to discipline Mat. Mat lived with his mother but went to visit his stepbrother at his father's home. It was only when all three members of the family could see how this dynamic was working that they could enter a reciprocal agreement in which all three had certain responsibilities. These were represented in the tasks which were agreed, and in the joint evaluations they conducted during the task-centred work (Portfolio D 2002: 5.1).

Two or more interlinked agreements might be appropriate when separate work is being undertaken, perhaps with a child and their parents, or with more than one household. Following separation and fresh partnerships, new families are created with important, but often difficult, relationships to each other. In these circumstances the interconnected but separate problems and goals might be reflected in different agreements, perhaps involving other professionals, too. In these circumstances it is important that everybody involved is aware of any other agreements, and that the reasons for having more than one agreement are understood.

TASKS

Task-centred practice derives its name from the central significance of the notion of task (see Chapter 2). The task is a vehicle which helps people take small steps towards something they want to achieve and, more than this, a means of entering another person's world. Developing and doing tasks as part of a systematic, shared strategy to achieving something bigger is, in itself, energising and empowering.

Options

Tasks are developed for completion between one session and the next, though some tasks may be completed within the session itself, rather like a workshop, and others may be repeated from one session to another. Usually there are no more than three tasks for each person, and some tasks may be mutual or reciprocal ('We will . . .'; 'J will . . . and K will . . .'). Ideas for future tasks might arise ('If we get to D, we'll be able to do E and F') but, by and large, there is no grand strategy mapping out tasks through the whole stretch of work; systematic though it is, task-centred practice is also opportunistic, and new openings will arise during the work itself. For example, the work with Evelyn was suddenly very successful, when she was offered a new tenancy as a result of her paying off considerable debts via the task-centred programme, and new tasks needed to respond quickly to this change (Portfolio G 2000).

Some ideas for tasks are likely to have featured in the earlier stages of the work when exploring problems and agreeing goals, though they will not have been formalised as 'tasks' as such. While what has and has not worked in the recent past is a guide to considering the development of tasks, the focus of the work is present and forward looking, so it is important to stimulate new thinking ('outside the box').

> Wayne and I discussed his drug misuse in greater depth and we reminded ourselves that the goal of becoming drug free is a massive undertaking as Wayne has experienced several years of addiction. Having discussed the psychological obstacles that Wayne needs to overcome we generated alternative ideas for achieving his goal by introducing new tasks.
>
> (Portfolio F 2003: 5.1)

As we will see in Chapter 7, the methods used to record the work can help this process of creative thinking, with many people finding a flipchart particularly freeing.

Generating tasks is not intended to be a test of creativity and it is just as effective to use tried and tested sets of tasks, such as those in Reid's (2000) task planners. Indeed, it would be excellent to see data banks of information available to practitioners to help guide future work by learning from present practice, as long as these were tailored to individual circumstances and not delivered as a package. Each encounter is unique, but it also has features in common with others. Since practitioners already act on these commonalities in implicit ways, all the better to make these explicit and build our bank of evidence-based practice.

Task planning and implementation

Reid and his colleagues have developed and researched a sequence for planning and implementing tasks which enhances task completion (Tolson *et al.* 1994; Reid 2000). A modified example of this is found in Box 6.6. Essentially, the sequence asks all those involved in the planning and implementation to consider what the task is, why do it and how to do it.

What is the task?

Tasks are chosen in order to help alleviate the selected problem and make progress to the related goal. The exploration of problems will have increased awareness of what resources have been or might be available, and the goal will have been framed with this in mind.

As we have seen, tasks should be chosen only after different task options have been considered. There are potentially many paths leading to the achievement of the goal, so it is important to leave the tramlines and open up alternatives, a process which can itself be pleasurable. It is one of the paradoxes of task-centred practice that its name should be associated with a word which is synonymous with chore, duty and work, and yet is experienced as so energising.

> The fact that she enjoyed the task that she set obviously went a long way towards motivating Sharon to complete it.
>
> (Portfolio A 2000: 5.2)

Once a task is agreed (which usually occurs after the questions of why and how have also been discussed), it is important that there is a lucid statement of it, usually written, to make sure everyone is really clear about the nature of the task and who it involves.

BOX 6.6: TASK PLANNING AND IMPLEMENTATION

- *Choosing the task*
  We used a flipchart to think of lots of different things I could do about this problem and Victoria (the worker) explained the process. We also looked at how these would help with the goal. I'd felt early on that I wanted to write things down about what it felt like, etc. so the first task we agreed came naturally.
- *Agreeing the task*
  We agreed four tasks. Task 1 was for me 'To write down what happens when I lose my temper with my son, Tom'. I hope this will help me to understand what leads up to this happening, what the effects are, etc.
- *Planning details*
  We discussed the details of how I would carry out the task, e.g. would I just write about a chosen number of incidents each week to provide a 'snapshot', or would I write up all incidents? Would I write them up immediately afterwards or at a pre-arranged time, eg in the evenings? I decided I wanted to write down all incidents, and would do this in the evenings when I've got more time.
- *Our commitment*
  I feel the benefits of the task will be to provide material for our sessions, and to look at situations from Tom's point of view. I am a 'diary' kind of person and I'm keen on this method of gathering information. A consequence of not doing this task could be overlooking some detail of what happens when I lose my temper with Tom. I feel Victoria is committed to helping me with this.
- *Possible obstacles*
  At first, no obstacles were anticipated, but once we'd discussed it in more detail, it became apparent that for me to write down details of every incident where I'd lost my temper would be a huge task. After discussion, I decided to write up every incident but only briefly, as a prompt to discussion and understanding in our next session.
- *Guidance*
  I don't feel I need to rehearse anything now with you, but I feel fine about sharing what I'm doing with my husband.
- *Task review*
  (Next session) see Chapter 7.

(based on Portfolio A 2000: 4.2)

Why this task?

An understanding of why the task has been agreed is central to enhancing commitment to it. A discussion of the benefits of successful completion and the possible consequences of neglecting the task is important, including how it links to the problem and the goal:

> Wayne and I discussed the long-term benefits of becoming drug free i.e. employment and educational opportunities, financial independence, forming a relationship etc. . . . Wayne was already stating his desire to stop using drugs but asking him to consider the potential outcome of achieving his goal helped to reinforce his desire.
>
> (Portfolio F 2003: 4.2)

The task-centred effort is designed to bring extra energies and resources to the situation, including the attention and strategic help of the practitioner. The process of generating options and agreeing tasks should feel liberating and continue to reinforce the partnership between those involved in the agreement. The impact of concerted attention cannot be underestimated and is reflected below in the reflections of a practitioner when working with a young man with learning difficulties moving into independent living:

> Dave did settle down to talking to me once he realised it was quite safe to talk to me about his feelings, but could not understand why anyone was interested in how he felt. I actually felt quite privileged that he had sat through the session.
>
> (Portfolio E 2000: 4.4)

How to do the task

Tasks need to be sufficiently stretching that they take people further than would have been possible without this work, but not so great that they falter. The best judge of this distance is the service user or carer, but only after they have been able to consider the task in detail and in context. Frequently, the detail of how a task will be done helps to reshape it, sometimes leading to a decision that what was considered one task is, in fact, many. A task such as 'to write down what happens when I lose my temper with my son, Tom' (Box 6.6) seems initially straightforward, but when the implementation is discussed in detail and in the context in which it will be completed, its complexity is revealed.

Coaching can improve the chances of a task being completed. This usually entails work in the session together, perhaps visualising the task being completed, rehearsing it or modelling it.

> Dave and I went through each step of the procedure [of using a photo booth] by putting a chair in front of his mirror to reproduce the situation in the photo booth.
>
> (Portfolio E 2000: 4.2)

One of the purposes of detailing the task is to anticipate possible obstacles. Just like the process of generating options for tasks, generating possible obstacles requires workers, users and carers to use their imagination and to think how some obstacles can be re-framed.

> Rather than asking, 'do you see any obstacles that might interfere with your success in completing this task?', this issue could be raised in other ways: 'what needs to happen for the task to be implemented successfully?'.
>
> (Caspi and Reid 2002: 265)

Kelly is agoraphobic and wants to be able to leave her house without panic. In her work with Kelly and her partner Tina, the practitioner helped to generate these potential obstacles to the completion of a task to go to the front door and open it:

> Someone may be at the door when I open it;
> someone may be walking along the corridor;
> the man opposite may be coming out of his flat;
> there may be workmen;
> Tina may be unwell and unable to accompany me.
>
> (Portfolio B 2002: 4.2)

Each of these possibilities can be assessed for their likelihood and Kelly and Tina can rehearse strategies to use if the potential obstacles become actual ones. Quite often, an analysis of obstacles will involve more contextual issues such as when and where the task is best attempted (see Boxes 6.7 and 6.8 and Activity 6.6).

Occasionally, the work generates more confidence in service users and carers than the worker feels is justified. It is always proper for the worker to express any realistic concerns they have, and to explain why an analysis of possible obstacles is important, but ultimately the task-centred method relies on trust.

> The main difficulty experienced in the development of tasks was John's enthusiasm . . . the stage that I found the least successful in the TPIS [Task Planning and Implementation Sequence] was the analysis of obstacles. The reason being that no matter how I tried to get John to discuss possible obstacles he refused.
>
> (Portfolio K 2002: 4.1; 4.2)

BOX 6.7: EXAMPLE OF TASKS: DAVE

Task	Task review	Rating
Task 1 (Dave) Have passport-size photos taken for bus pass	See Chapter 7 for reviewing tasks	See Chapter 7
Task 2 (Kathy – worker) Fill out bus pass application form, have signed by boss		

Task 1 notes

Dave will need three £1 coins.
Dave to go to town to the photo booth in the bus station – ensured Dave knew where the bus station is and the whereabouts of the booth.
To go into the booth and have photographs taken – we talked through the sequence.
If any difficulty using the booth to ask for assistance from the office.
Dave to take the photographs to the office to obtain the bus pass for next week's hospital appointment.
Kathy reassured Dave that if he could not manage the task, that we would look at other ways of obtaining the photographs.

(Portfolio E 2000: 4.1)

BOX 6.8: EXAMPLE OF TASKS: WAYNE

Task	Task review	Rating
Task 1 (Wayne) Wayne will explain to his sister that he is going to try to stop using heroin and that he will not be visiting her home until he feels able to be around her when she is using heroin.	See Chapter 7 for reviewing tasks	See Chapter 7
Task 2 (Wayne) Wayne will ensure that he's out of bed and dressed for 2 p.m. Thu. in order to be available for appointment with specialist drugs worker.		
Task 3 (Barbara – worker) Barbara will refer Wayne to specialist drugs worker and provide details of Wayne's drug misuse history and current legal status.		
Task 4 (Barbara) Barbara will talk to Wayne's mum about the support that he will need over the next few weeks.		

(Portfolio F 2003: 4.1)

ACTIVITY 6.6: TRAINER

Developing an understanding of tasks and task development

- What use could you make of the two examples of agreed tasks (Boxes 6.7 and 6.8) to develop learners' understanding of how to develop tasks with 'built-in' success?
- How could the components of Task Planning and Implementation (Box 6.6) be used in conjunction with these examples of agreed tasks to further learners' understanding?

Who should suggest and do tasks?

The task-centred work is a partnership and, as such, it relies on each person playing their part. When it is going well it is often difficult to remember quite who suggested which task, because it arose out of the discussion and was shaped and reshaped in subsequent talk. Workers, users and carers alike may find the 'imagination muscle' hard to locate early in the work, but will discover that the exercise of generating options for tasks and imagining obstacles can become second nature with practice. Research suggests that it is unimportant who originates a task, as long as the planning and implementation elements are thoroughly considered (Reid 1997).

> Evelyn did really well when we brainstormed what needed to be done and found it helpful when these task were written down and prioritised. I felt a real sense of working together in this as the tasks I suggested, such as contacting schools, GP, etc. [about the move], she had not thought about.
>
> (Portfolio G 2000: 4.2)

The idea of partnership suggests a balance of tasks between parties in the agreement, even though 'sometimes it is much easier to make choices or carry out an action on behalf of the service user instead of encouraging them to participate' (Portfolio K 2002: 2.1). One worker had been concerned how many tasks the user had to do, but at the next session it transpired she had managed very well and told the worker that she had 'just worked her way through the list'. A general principle is that when a service user or carer can undertake a task, they should. However, there are tasks which more naturally fall to the worker because of their role and access to resources:

> I [social worker] agreed to arrange with Dr Jennings to begin outpatients 15 minutes early so Kelly may see the doctor when the waiting room is empty.
>
> (Portfolio B 2002: 4.3)

We have noted several times that the process of task-centred work is systematic but not linear. This is true of task development and implementation. Frequently, this process will throw new light on the problem, help to refine and readjust the goal, perhaps suggest new parties to the agreement:

> Although we were just working with Evelyn at this stage, I suggested to her that it may be helpful to include Carl [her son] in the work if he was willing.
>
> (Portfolio G 2000: 4.1)

Once the pattern of task development is established, people become familiar with it and the workings of this stage of the model, and they often become quite adept at modifying it. Increasingly, people exercise choices based on knowledge and experience of their problems, their goals and the way task-centred practice works:

> Task:
>
> Kelly, Tina and Erica [the social worker] to go downstairs in the lift and, if Kelly is well enough, to try and stand outside the front door.
>
> We acknowledged that this task is potentially two separate tasks and hence Kelly has more chance of it being successful. She can choose to complete less of it and remain with a sense of achievement and her confidence intact and if she feels able she can achieve more, then it is the next step.

> Kelly opted for the sessional tasks to be a step ahead of the homework tasks.
>
> (Portfolio B 2002: 4.1)

Sometimes workers can feel inhibited about involving other people because of their own ideas about how this might be interpreted by the client, but it is always wise to check this out:

> Dan felt he may have greater success in completing these tasks if his mother knew of the tasks and was able to encourage and support him in completing them. I had also thought of this but had held back from suggesting it as I did not want Dan to feel I had no faith in him completing the goals alone.
>
> (Portfolio L 2000: 4.1)

In Chapter 7 we consider the next stages of task-centred working: reviewing tasks and evaluating the work. We will also consider the central role of making a record of the work jointly with service users and carers.

KEY POINTS

- ☐ It is important to appreciate the *context* of practice.
- ☐ The task-centred process aims to move *towards* partnership; the speed and degree of success will vary enormously from one situation to another.
- ☐ Task-centred practice focuses on the here and now.
- ☐ Practitioners should avoid giving solutions; working on one's own chosen goal is an important experience of self-determination.
- ☐ Tasks are central to the journey from problem to goal, but task-centred work is also *person-centred.*
- ☐ The Task Planning and Implementation Sequence has been found to increase the success rate for task completion.

KEY READING

Doel, M. and Marsh, P. (1992) *Task-centered Social Work* Aldershot, UK: Ashgate

The first comprehensive account of task-centred practice for the UK context was Doel and Marsh's (1992) *Task-centred Social Work*. The authors may be biased, but we hope this remains a useful introduction to task-centred work!

Reid, W. J. (2000) *The Task Planner: An Intervention Resource for Human Service Planners* New York: Columbia University Press

This is a thorough and well-researched compilation of task strategies, presented in alphabetical order (Alcoholism/Addiction, Anger Management . . . right through to Withdrawn Child). It is entirely US in derivation, but still useful for UK and other contexts.

Trevithick, P. (2000) *Social Work Skills* Buckingham: Open University Press.

This has become a classic and is an exceptionally useful all-round text for the skills of social work practice, to set alongside the specifically task-centred skills explored in this one, *The Task-Centred Book*.

CHAPTER 7

REVIEW

OBJECTIVES

By the end of this chapter you should:

- Understand the purpose of review
- Know how to conduct a review of tasks
- Be able to use a self-rating scale for task completion, and enable others to use it
- Relate task review to problem alleviation and goal achievement
- Evaluate the overall impact of task-centred work.

THE PURPOSE OF REVIEW

Review, literally 'to see again', has many dictionary definitions, the two most relevant to our purposes being 'examining something to make sure that it is adequate, accurate, or correct', and 'to re-examine something, to take another look at or consideration of something' (Encarta 1999). In the task-centred model, there is also a technical meaning with reference to 'task review', which we explore in detail later in this chapter. Evaluation, a notion closely linked to review, is a term we reserve for a more formal review of the whole of the task-centred experience, usually as part of the final session, and we consider this towards the end of this chapter.

A review should focus on both the outcomes and the processes of the work. A review of *outcomes* considers current progress towards the goal, how the tasks are helping (or not) to achieve change, and the impact this is having on the selected problems. One of the major purposes is, therefore, to check that the tasks are doing what they are supposed to, i.e. helping people move towards their goals and alleviating the problems. The review enables participants to reconsider the selected problem. Is it proving to be the right choice? The goal, too, may be reviewed, to discuss whether it needs any redefinition or whether there are other people who should be involved in the agreement.

> At this initial stage I feel it is becoming apparent that there will be need for two agreements to be drawn up. Possibly between Diana and Mat [mother and son], and Daniel and Mat [stepbrothers].
>
> (Portfolio D 2002: 2.2)

A review of *processes* focuses on the means which have been used to achieve the outcomes. This will entail a discussion of feelings about the experience of the work, and the value and meaning of the work so far. Reviewing the processes helps everyone to understand the way the task-centred model works, so the review process has an expressive function as well as a cognitive one. The review is a time to take stock; how was this task experienced, how did these behaviours change as a result of those actions? Everyone learns from the activity of reviewing, and the review itself helps to consolidate this learning, with the aim of generalising it to other situations yet to be experienced.

Reviews of outcomes and processes are both equally important. If we take a journey as a metaphor, the review of outcomes figures out how far we have gone and how near we are to the destination (and is this still the best route?), whereas the review of process is to check how people are feeling, whether anyone has car sickness and wants a break, someone else wants a turn at the wheel, and everyone feels that they have been included in the 'map-reading'. If the journey itself is being experienced poorly, changes need to be agreed.

> With regards to success or failure, John felt he had done well to attempt all the tasks set, but was a little disappointed with the way he had *felt* while carrying them out.
>
> (Portfolio K 2002: 4.3 – our emphasis)

Another purpose of a review is to consider the question of *timing*. The review may renew the substance of the agreement (problem, goal, range of tasks, etc.), but reveal the need for a rescheduling. Perhaps progress has been interrupted by unforeseen events; perhaps the goal is likely to be achieved earlier or later than first anticipated. The time limit was decided relatively early in the work, and was a 'guesstimate'. Firm deadlines are key to the momentum which sustains the work, but flexibility is needed if circumstances are so changed that the original deadline is no longer feasible.

The alliance

Reviewing the work builds and strengthens the alliance between people. Like working on a jigsaw puzzle together, there is a shared commitment to completing the final picture; each spends some time separately examining certain pieces and other times, heads are down together, working together on another piece. Each person is involved in the same process of task development, enactment and review; the review, in particular, increases the sense of mutual responsibility. When family members are all involved in an agreement, with perhaps a combination of individual, reciprocal and mutual tasks, this alliance can be all the stronger. Successes are better enjoyed when they can be celebrated together, and when things are difficult and tasks have not been achieved, the support which this alliance offers enables the participants to learn from the experience and try again, either with the unsuccessful task or with a new one.

One of the purposes of reviews is to strengthen this alliance. The review should lead to an honest reassessment of the situation in a blame-free way. Regular reviews of progress will make any difficulties explicit, and provide a systematic framework to examine why and what is needed.

> Evaluating the process makes the worker more accountable.
>
> (Portfolio A 2000: 5.2)

This alliance carries responsibilities which hold workers accountable to service users and carers. As we explored in Chapter 6, this does not mean that workers always do what service users and carers want them to do, nor does it mean that workers abdicate their professional authority. On the contrary, accountability cannot be separated from openness about the professional's authority and issues of power. Where there are disagreements between workers and service users or carers, being accountable means giving a clear and honest account of what the disagreement is and why, and the review provides a stage for this.

Accountability in task-centred practice is more commonly about workers, service users and carers all being able to give an account of their part in the work. Regular reviewing of the work is the way in which this account can be maintained (see Activity 7.1). We will see later in this chapter how task-centred recording reinforces this accountability.

ACTIVITY 7.1: PRACTITIONER

Reviews and task-centred practice

- In what ways does the function of review in task-centred practice differ from the reviews you currently undertake in your work?
- What aspects of the review in task-centred work would fit best with your current practice and which would need adaptation? What kinds of adaptation would be possible?

REVIEWING TASKS

Let us remind ourselves in a figure of how the task review stage fits into the overall sequence of the model (Figure 7.1).

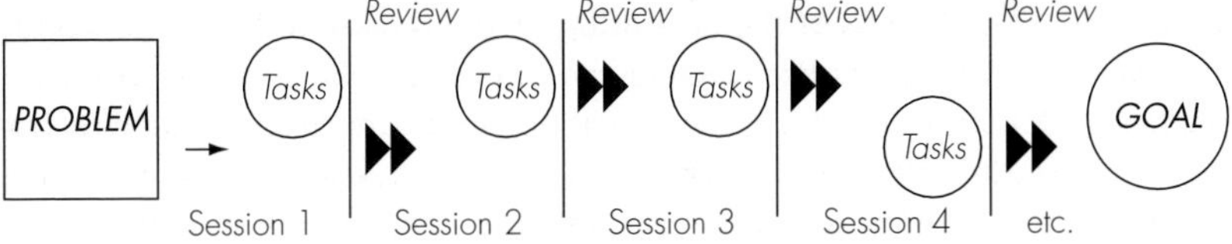

FIGURE 7.1 Task review within the overall model

Figure 7.1 is a little simplified, so in Figure 7.2 we consider a section in more detail.

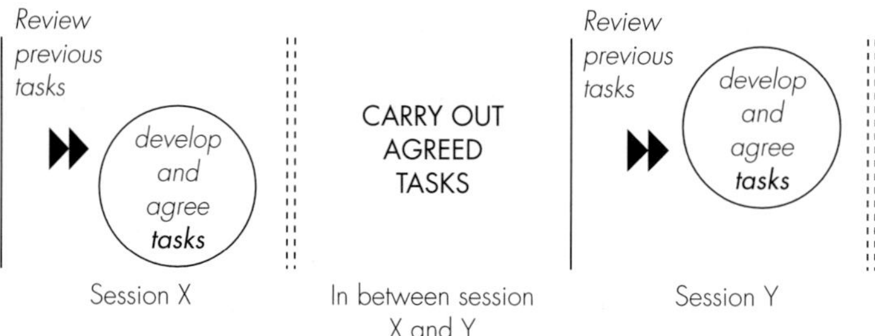

FIGURE 7.2 Task review and task work

What is missing from Figure 7.1 is the time in between each session, in which people carry out their tasks. Some tasks may, of course, be completed in the session itself (sessional tasks) and these often involve some coaching or rehearsal, but most tasks are likely to be completed in the time between one session and another. Success is more likely if the specifics of a task, such as timing, are determined through discussion; for example, 'Suzy will meet Jim at the bus stop at five o'clock on Monday and Wednesday of the coming week'.

Once the first set of tasks have been developed (usually in the first or second session of the work), the following session begins with a review of the tasks which were agreed at the previous session and carried out during the period between then and now. So, as Reid (1992: 66) notes, 'tasks are generally reviewed toward the beginning of each session'. Of course, it is important to follow social conventions around welcome and settling in, but the worker should avoid an invitation to start talking about the situation in a general way, such as 'how's it going?'. Similarly, if the service user or carer drifts into what is in fact the matter for the review, the practitioner should either suggest a pause, or move into the task review format. So, the service user perhaps says, 'I've got lots to tell you about what's been going on – you'll never guess how it went with Cameron . . . '; the worker should pick up on the tone and feelings, such as 'I can see we're going to have lots to talk about, and it's sounding good', but suggest a process, such as 'but are you OK if we do this a step at a time? It's just that it will help us to make sure we cover everything and don't miss anything out. Is that OK?'.

As each session passes, everyone will become familiar with the pattern of welcome and settling in, structured review of work on tasks, learning from this to develop new tasks (using the Task Planning and Implementation Sequence in Chapter 6) and summarising the tasks which have been agreed to be completed between now and the next session.

Of course, the pattern is never quite so dry and linear. Much will depend on how the tasks have gone, so the review is crucial in setting the scene for the session as a whole. There might be some edginess at the beginning of the session as everyone wonders how successful task completion has been. Sometimes there may have been a crisis which has blown the tasks off course, in which case it will be important to spend time reviewing the nature of the crisis and offering any appropriate support. At some point, when everyone is able to refocus, it is important to return to the task-centred agreement to discuss together what is to be done with it; has it been merely postponed or have the new circumstances fundamentally altered its relevance?

Process of task review

The process of task review is systematic but not mechanical. At every opportunity it is important that everyone is reminded about the wider significance of the tasks, i.e. their key role in helping to achieve the goal. Reminders of the rewards which achievement of the goal will bring (motivational, practical, physical, etc.) are also helpful. Therefore, the task review will almost always include a consideration of the selected problem (how are the tasks helping to reduce it?) and the goal (how are the tasks taking people nearer?).

Everyone should have a copy of the tasks as they were written down at the last session and it is important that everyone involved has their own copy to refer to between sessions (see the section on Recording later in this chapter). Sometimes the tasks may have been recorded on a flipchart left with the service user or carer, with the worker making their own copy. Carbonated recording pads enable at least three copies to be available, one for the service user and carer, one for the worker and one for the agency record. Tasks need to have been recorded so that there is space to the right of each to record the review, and another smaller space for the rating (see Boxes 7.1 and 7.2).

Each task is discussed in turn. What was the experience of working on the task and was it completed as planned? If it was largely successful, this should be celebrated, especially if it required effort, courage or ingenuity. Were there aspects of the task which had not been anticipated and which needed quick thinking or action? What has been learned from this successful experience and how can this be used to develop new tasks? In the current jargon, there is a search for the drivers (see Box 7.3).

If the task is not attempted or only minimally achieved, it is just as important to consider what happened and why. Before turning to identify the obstacles, the worker should express support, just in case there are any fears that continuing involvement is seen as contingent on success. Before moving to an analysis of what went wrong and why, time should be spent acknowledging any feelings, such as disappointment, anger, frustration or embarrassment. Finding out what obstacles prevented the success of the task and doing this without blame or guilt, can be a new experience for some people. Indeed, the learning from a task which was not completed can sometimes be greater than successful completion and is usually an opportunity to rethink. When Evelyn failed to bring a list of what she had spent her money on over the previous week, the worker turned this into a sessional task, and they worked together on outgoings and income, which proved very illuminating for Evelyn (Portfolio G 2000: 4.3). This same worker reflected on how this task had seemed straightforward, but was not:

> I felt that this was a relatively simple task, specific, within Evelyn's control and time-limited, all positive indicators for achievement. On reflection, this task did take some effort and I felt there was a lack of commitment and motivation on Evelyn's part . . . I had not taken account of Evelyn's disorganised and chaotic lifestyle and that to actually sit down and record all her spending would be very difficult for her. Although I felt a sense of frustration at first that the task had not been successful, I subsequently wondered if the task set was not the right one, particularly as Evelyn had had debt counselling in the past.
>
> (Portfolio G 2000: 4.3)

Failed tasks can provide a useful prompt 'to a consideration of obstacles and related options' (Reid 1992: 66). A careful, forensic approach is needed to discover exactly what

BOX 7.1: EXAMPLE TASK REVIEW: WAYNE

Task	Task review	Rating
Task 1 (Wayne) Wayne will ignore arguments between his younger sisters and will not get involved. He will either go to his bedroom to avoid them or go for a walk.	*Task 1 review* Wayne had managed to do this on every occasion. He had not been involved in a verbal altercation with his sisters all week.	*Rating* 5 positive success
Task 2 (Wayne) Wayne will say 'hello' to the neighbours when he next sees them in the garden. If he finds them to be approachable, he will apologise for shouting at them when they had their car radio on last week.	*Task 2 review* Wayne was not able to undertake this task, he still felt very angry towards his neighbours and thought that any approach might start an argument.	*Rating* 0 not attempted
Task 3 (Barbara – worker) Barbara will find out about local self-defence classes which run in the area. These will allow Wayne to burn up some physical energy and feel more confident and assertive when challenged.	*Task 3 review* Barbara brought leaflets and telephone numbers of a variety of social sporting activities that Wayne might pursue.	*Rating* 5 positive success

(Portfolio F 2003: 4.3)

happened and why; in particular, whether the obstacles were mainly ones of opportunity, inadequate task preparation, insufficient detail in planning, misunderstanding, psychological barriers such as motivation or fear, or a combination of these and other factors. It is useful to revisit the Task Planning and Implementation Sequence (Chapter 6) to review the difficulties which have been experienced with a failed task (see Activity 7.2).

BOX 7.2: EXAMPLE OF TASK REVIEW: MRS SARITA AND MR HILL

Task	Task review	Rating
Task 1 (Mrs S and Mr H) Mrs Sarita and Mr Hill to avoid getting into arguments with Yusef by saying 'I don't want to argue with you' and, if necessary, walking away.	*Task 1 review* Some arguments had been avoided by using this approach, but there had been other occasions when Mr Hill got into arguments with Yusef because Yusef was good at winding Mr Hill up.	*Rating* 3 partial success
Task 2 (Mrs S and Mr H) Mrs Sarita and Mr Hill to support one another in letting Yusef know what's right and what's wrong.	*Task 2 review* On some occasions they had supported one another, but not on others (e.g. Mr Hill took Yusef's bike away as a punishment, but then Mrs Sarita allowed Yusef to go out on it later).	*Rating* 2 limited success
Task 3 (Mrs S and Mr H) Mrs Sarita and Mr Hill to praise Yusef when he is good.	*Task 3 review* There had been only one opportunity to praise Yusef for good behaviour in the last week.	*Rating* 2 limited success

(Portfolio H 1996: 4.3)

ACTIVITY 7.2: LEARNER

Reviewing a failed task

In the first example Task Review sheet (Box 7.1), Wayne says that he did not attempt Task 2 and gives himself a zero rating.

How would you review this task in order to help Wayne and yourself learn the most from it?

BOX 7.3: EXAMPLE OF TASK REVIEW NOTES: DAVE

Task 1 (Dave) Obtaining photographs Rating *5*

I asked how Dave felt the task went.

Took longer than expected. He was nervous and did not complete the task at the first attempt. He went back the following week because he did not want to let me [worker] down.

I asked Dave how he felt now the task had been completed.

He felt proud when the task was completed, he did not expect to be able to do it. He was anxious it took longer than agreed – I reassured him it did not matter, the outcome was good.

(Portfolio E 2000: 4.3)

The self-rating system (Box 7.4) is one which people use to score their own progress on each task (including workers' rating their own task achievement). Practitioners sometimes feel uncomfortable asking people to score themselves, feeling a bit like 'teacher', especially if the task has been poorly accomplished. However, it is worth practising the self-rating because it often leads to further useful discussion which throws light on issues of self-belief. Sometimes success is hard to recognise or accept and it is not unusual, especially early in the task-centred work, for a person to give themself a lower rating than the practitioner would estimate. Ultimately, the rating belongs to the person whose task is being reviewed, but it is right to share any perception that the task completion is being under-rated (or, less commonly, over-rated).

> Dan was not always comfortable with the idea of a 'rating' and tended to go with the 'all or nothing' approach (0 or 5). However, the ratings were often modified after discussion. For example, the 'Dan will begin to tidy his bedroom' task was initially a zero, as he had not done anything in practical terms. However, once we began to explore the task it became obvious that it was extremely non-specific and this had been unhelpful as Dan had not

BOX 7.4: SELF-RATING TASK COMPLETION

Scale

5 = complete success
4 = substantial success
3 = some success
2 = partial success
1 = no success
0 = not attempted

(or other words which convey this scale)

> known 'where to start'. Dan had thought hard about the task during the week and had begun to break it down ready to offer suggestions for tasks in the following session. After discussion we decided this activity in itself deserved a rating of 1. Again, my role was in highlighting the positives.
>
> (Portfolio L 2000: 4.3)

Behaviour can change before awareness of change. In other words, recognition of new behaviours may only slowly emerge from the shadow of an enduring difficulty. It can take time to appreciate that positive changes are actually occurring, and the self-rating system can accelerate this process (see Activity 7.3).

> Task Review:
> Evelyn did speak to Carl [her son] when he asked her for money, and she had not lent him any. She had explained why and asked him to look at ways he could save money for himself. Although Evelyn thought this 'hadn't done any good', Carl had now bought a half-fare bus pass and was giving her £15 per week housekeeping money as soon as his benefit money arrived.
>
> (Portfolio G 2000: 4.3)

ACTIVITY 7.3: MANAGER

Task-centred reviews and agency review systems

- In what ways does the notion of review in task-centred practice fit with current systems of review in your agency?
- What, if any, advantages does the task-centred review have for accountability and partnership working in your agency?
- How might the task-centred review process and those which already exist in the agency be integrated?

The bigger picture

> John stated, 'I have wanted to do this for such a long time but kept putting it off because it felt like such a big thing'.
>
> (Portfolio K 2002: 5.1)

As well as the detailed review of work on tasks, which we consider shortly, a review is an opportunity to stand back and reflect on the bigger picture. As such, it is an essential part of the task-centred work for everyone involved. John (above) suddenly realises a wish that would not have been possible before his worker helped him find confidence.

Practitioners will need to review their own work, too. The bigger picture for practitioners concerns their own practice development. If they are relatively inexperienced, they will wish to check out their use of the model, especially as they adapt it to their own style and setting – how 'task-centred' is it? More experienced task-centred practitioners will be keen to consider how their experience of this particular example of task-centred work contrasts with past ones, and what new learning they have derived from it. Full awareness of other people's worlds might come only when practitioners have the chance to review their work:

> On reflection Wayne was pressured by me to carry out Task 2 [Box 7.1] and I failed to spot his reluctance. His lack of motivation and fear of confrontation in speaking to his neighbours made him unlikely to carry out the task . . .
>
> . . . Wayne had grown up in a family that was totally dependent upon the state benefit system. For him, finding employment was a long-shot and in any event would create a situation where his mother's level of benefit would be affected, thus creating the 'cycle of deprivation' or 'underclass'. The most realistic option for Wayne was to add to the family's income in a way that was non means tested – illegal activity.
>
> My discussion with Wayne about employment or training at times felt both patronising and unrealistic.
>
> (Portfolio F 2003: 4.3; 4)

Of course, any new insights from this opportunity to review practice needs to be taken back into the direct work with service users and carers.

Gathering evidence for a task-centred portfolio is a constant form of review for practitioners, and it is important to support continuing professional development (via special interest groups, for instance) even when the formal work on the portfolio is finished. Supervisors and managers have a significant role to play, either by participating directly in reviews of task-centred practice, or by encouraging learning organisations in which this kind of continuing professional development is a regular feature.

By taking a step to one side, practitioners learn more about the people they are working with, about themselves, their practice and their assumptions. In her work with Evelyn, the worker realised that it did not take too many 'slips' for a person's life to become seriously difficult. She visited the day before Evelyn's move to a new flat to find her in tears because the friend of a friend who said he would help her move had let her down. The worker's doubts about this arrangement were confirmed, and she was able to make other arrangments for Evelyn at the last minute. Similarly, the worker discovered that Evelyn had not thought to consider whether the new property had a gas supply (for her gas cooker); at the worker's suggestion Evelyn did make enquiries and discovered that there was no gas connection, so the worker arranged a loan to purchase a new electric cooker. It is easy to see how poor judgement about others' reliability, and difficulty in anticipating problems in an increasingly complex environment, can lead to a spiral of problems which, in Evelyn's case, had led to her three children being taken temporarily into public care (Portfolio G 2000: 4.2).

Practitioners are encouraged by the review process in task-centred practice to consider how the method is working and to undertake regular critical appraisals of their practice (see Activity 7.4).

> I am not sure at this stage of the work [end of problem exploration] whether the selected problem is concise enough to inform further work. If not, perhaps this points to my skill as a practitioner in eliciting enough information and detail from the client and using this constructively, and may be it's something I need to address later.
>
> (Portfolio A 2000: 2.3)

ACTIVITY 7.4: SUPERVISOR

Reviewing a practitioner's task-centred work

Kumlaish is an experienced task-centred practitioner and completed a post-qualifying task-centred practice portfolio two years ago.

As Kumlaish's supervisor, what part do you see yourself playing in helping her to undertake regular reviews of her task-centred work? What would this look like in practice?

RECORDING TASK-CENTRED WORK

> He said that by writing [the problems] down in this way they did not seem as daunting as when he just thought about them in his head.
>
> (Portfolio F 2003: 2.2)

Keeping a record of work is essential to good practice and usually necessary to fulfil agency and legal requirements (Department of Health 2000, 2002). However, recording systems which are devised *for* people rather than *with* them are more likely to be written, framed and stored in ways which are not easily accessible to them. Even though most systems profess that they have service users' and carers' interests at heart, the way in which they are developed and put into operation frequently does not include piloting them.

The drive to ensure that professional shall speak unto professional is in danger of forgetting that the first duty is to speak unto service user and carer. Integrated information for health and social care has generated single assessment documents which are often tick-box and massive. Rather than relying on an open question such as 'Where would you like to go on holiday?', these single assessment packages rely on the 'To which of the following fifty countries would you like to go on holiday?'. Apart from the laborious nature of this style of questioning, it also misses the fact that the question might not allow the person to focus on the significant aspect for them ('I'm not bothered about the country, but I do want to be near the sea'). Indeed, it was reported that

> workers found [the single assessment tools] were rather like market research and somewhat fragmented in their approach . . . therefore vital information had to be recorded separately. Because of the length of time it took to complete and the amount of questions that had to be covered, clients became agitated and at time confused.
>
> (Unpublished project for the Advanced Award in Social Work)

Two hours was the average length of time reported in this study to complete the single assessment document.

All task-centred recording is 'piloted' with users and carers because it takes place interactively with them. The process of recording task-centred work is closely integrated with the work itself, with workers using shared recording methods with people. Practitioners often find that they are recording in quite different ways when using task-centred methods, mainly because the record is completed *in situ* rather than with hindsight back at the office.

> The initial stages of recording with the family I found uncomfortable, my usual method of recording would be back at the office and signed off by my line manager. . . . As the task-centred process progressed this became easier and a natural part of the work.
>
> (Portfolio D 2002: 5.3)

The task-centred method encourages the use of graphic recording methods, most notably flipcharts. A number of practitioners have remarked that the visibility of a flipchart to all concerned means more ownership of the work, and the possibility to check things out more carefully. It keeps a curb on the use of language, too, so that people's own words are more likely to be recorded (see Box 7.5). It is not just a question of avoiding jargon, but of actively using people's own words and meanings. For example, as part of the task-centred work one parent had decided that it would be important for her to praise her son for the absence of poor behaviour, which she described as 'nothingness of behaviour'. To

BOX 7.5: EXAMPLE OF FLIPCHART NOTES: WAYNE

Problems

BASHING MY GUMS AT PEOPLE
Strangers, Neighbours, Family,
Shouting, Threatening, Swearing,
Hitting, Pushing, Prodding, Kicking

GOING ON THE ROB

Money, Handbags, Cars, Stereos, TV's,
Family, Friends, Strangers, Neighbours + shops,
Daily, Weekly, Monthly, Day time, night time – risk of going back to prison

USING HEROIN

Smoking, <u>Never injecting,</u> with Danny,
At home, At mates
£10 bag everyday or street methadone

NOT SLEEPING

All night – Using Heroin,
Go to bed at about 5am,
Can't get up for appointments,
Don't want to get up,
Don't want to go to bed,
Not tired

(Portfolio F 2003: 2.2; 5.3)

anybody outside this piece of task-centred work, this phrase would be meaningless, but its sense arose from the context of this work, and it was one which the service user had generated herself. Accordingly, the worker used it in her records and discussion (Portfolio A 2000: 4.3).

Important observations can be lost in ordinary discussion, and the flipchart helps to chart these issues by slowing down the process. Perhaps most important of all, this slowing helps people to make connections by graphically portraying relationships and associations (between people, between problems and tasks, between actions and consequences, etc.). Starting with a blank sheet of paper, a flipchart builds up a picture in which the complexity of people's situations can be faithfully represented, yet in a way which can increase confidence that something can be done.

> The technique of Mat [an 11-year-old] and Diana [his mother] being able to put their problems on the flipchart worked well in two ways: firstly it gave them a sense of ownership, that this was their work, and [second], both Diana and Mat were able to identify a connection in feelings, actions and responses.
>
> (Portfolio D 2002: 2.2)

Of course, it is important to be sensitive to issues of literacy and visual impairment, both of which will put some limitation on flipcharting and written record formats. Whatever is recorded needs to be accessible. Work with blind and visually impaired people might suggest the use of audiorecording. A flipchart can be useful for people with some vision, and because it lends itself to graphic, pictorial representations, this can also help non-readers to capture the discussion and decisions taken.

> As Kelly's literacy was quite poor I initially completed a written map for her as she was disclosing. This was useful so that I could recall specific details and to ensure that Kelly, Tina [Kelly's carer] and I were all armed with the same information. I felt that Kelly was potentially disadvantaged by so much writing and when I checked this out with her she agreed. Hence we developed picture graphics and we were each able to use this as a basis for our work.
>
> (Portfolio B 2002: 2.3)

In a review of her task-centred recording, one worker who did not use flipchart regretted a missed opportunity:

> In the future I would attempt to do the written recording on a large sheet of paper with marker pens to enable John to feel even more involved in the process. I may even encourage him to do a little of the recording himself so he really feels the work is designed by him and for him. The reason this was not done in this way to start with is due to the fact that I felt embarrassed to do so, knowing that this was *my* first experience of using task-centred social work and that my knowledge was limited.
>
> (Portfolio K 2002: 2.2 – our emphasis)

It may be that electronic packages will offer the same instant and interactional possibilities as we have discussed here, such as Liquidlogic and assessment kits like *Easycare* (www.sheffield.ac.uk/sisa/easycare; Wilson 2002), with the advantage that they do not need copying out again to be transported back to the workplace. Nevertheless, it is likely that the large format of a flipchart will continue to perform well.

EVALUATING THE WORK AS A WHOLE

One dictionary defines evaluate as 'to consider or examine something in order to judge its value, quality, importance, extent or condition' (Encarta 1999). Though similar to the notion of review, an evaluation focuses more on a judgement made about value. The final evaluation with service users and carers is, therefore, not just a review of outcomes and processes, but also an overall assessment of the value and impact of the experience as a whole. Returning to the metaphor of the journey which we used in relation to review, the evaluation is a time to consider whether the journey was worth the effort, did it take people where they wanted to be and is it a journey they would recommend to others? Have there been any spin-off benefits or any unforeseen dangers? And what do bystanders have to say about what they have witnessed? The evaluation includes judgements about the relative merit of this part of the journey over that part, and this mode of transport over that. In short, an evaluation is an opportunity for feedback, sometimes formalised via a questionnaire and the use of a scale to weigh the responses.

Outcomes and processes

The questions in Box 7.6 take people through a suggested sequence which starts with an evaluation of outcomes and moves to a consideration of processes in the work together. Box 7.7 is an alternative user evaluation format which can also be used at the conclusion of the work. The obvious outcome is the goal, but before turning attention to this aspect, the method systematically considers the original problems. To what extent has the selected problem been resolved and with hindsight, was this the right problem to have focused on? It is unlikely that there will be any surprises at this stage, since these issues will have been reviewed from time to time during the work. However, the ending of the work is a chance for people to exercise 'long sight' on the situation, with the focus on learning for future problem-solving.

A key consideration of the final evaluation is, of course, whether the goal has been achieved. After all, this is what everyone has been working towards. There may be a number of perspectives on this issue, but the most important is the service user's or carer's, since it is *their* goal.

> Sharon said she had come a long way towards achieving the goal as she was losing her temper less frequently and with less intensity than before. However, it wasn't completely resolved as there are still occasions when Sharon feels she loses her temper unnecessarily.
>
> (Portfolio A 2000: 5.1)

Sharon's 'good in parts' evaluation is not unusual. The degree of success is important, but seems less so than the fact that there has been *some* success, so it is the sensation of movement in the right direction, and the continuing momentum which this generates, that is experienced as highly positive. Moreover, there are frequently other results from the work which could not necessarily have been foreseen, yet are felt to be significant. For example, as a result of the task-centred programme, 16-year-old Carl started to give his mother £15 from his own benefits money as soon as it arrived and he also bought a half-fare bus pass which saved the family income (Portfolio G 2000: 4.3). These unforeseen consequences of the work need to be noted, even if they were not part of the plan.

BOX 7.6: EXAMPLE OF SERVICE USER'S EVALUATION: WAYNE

Q1 Are the selected problems the ones which you most wanted help with?
Yes, I needed to stop nicking or I was gonna get locked up again . . . I don't fight in the house as much now, my temper was way out of control, I needed to stop that . . . The heroin has been a big, big problem for a long time now and it won't go away that easy! I really wanted to stop.

Q2 If not, what is the problem which you would have liked help with?
Nothing else, these were enough weren't they?

Q3 How much of the original goal do you think has been achieved? Can you rate this 1–10?
I suppose I would score it at about 6 . . . Well, I haven't got kicked out of my mam's yet, 'cos I've been better with my sisters and the neighbours and I haven't got locked up for anything . . .
I'll do the drugs rattle in my own time, I've done it before so I can do it again. I thought I could do it but it was too hard. . . .
I haven't got a job 'cos I need to sort the drugs out first.

Q4 How much of the original goal do other people think you have achieved?
My mam's glad I've stopped going on the rob, she wants the neighbours to think we're alright, having just moved here.
Our Siobhan's glad that I couldn't do the heroin thing 'cos she'd be on her own doing it. My mam's glad I can't get a job 'cos she would be worse off.

Q5 What do you think about this way of working? (I clarified what this meant)
Funny, I'm not used to it, it's better than you just telling me to do it I suppose. It made me not want to let you down because you really seemed to want me to do it, but I suppose it's me I've let down, innit?

(At this point we discussed the positive progress that Wayne had made).

Q6 How do you feel about coping in the future now the agreement has ended?
OK, I'll do the heroin thing, my mam will help me and I'll just have to rattle . . . I'll be able to control my temper more, my sisters know that I don't get wound up so easy now.

Wayne agreed to continue to receive help from Paul, the specialist drugs worker.

(Portfolio F 2003: 5.1)

The evaluation also needs to concern the processes of the work together because the experience of the work is as significant as the outcome. The feedback from people as reported in practitioners' portfolios is mainly very positive and though we are relying on the accuracy of the workers' observations, there seems no reason to doubt this.

The brief extracts from practitioners' portfolios later in Box 7.8 give an indication of the value of the task-centred process, together with some of the reservations. In particular, they indicate the intricate layers of evaluation, which in addition to the 'How was it for you?' type, also encompass an assessment of the model of practice itself. Sometimes this can involve everyone, at other times it may just be part of the practitioners' dialogue with themselves (see Chapter 5).

BOX 7.7: EXAMPLE OF SERVICE USER'S EVALUATION: SHARON

These questions are asked because I would like you to let me know what you think about the work we have done together, and to help me to improve my work. This will help us both to get the best out of the ending of our work.

- *The beginning*
  Looking back to the beginning of our work, why do you think I got involved with you?

  To try and help me get a better understanding and not get trapped into negative habits.

- *Our written agreement*
  What did you think about our written agreement? Did you like this style of work? For example, did it help to use pens and paper in our work together?

  I think it is important to have a written agreement so that there is a focus and you can know whether you are getting anywhere.

- *The goal*
  How near to your goal are you? What tells you how near you are to your goal? How near to your goal do other people think you are?

  I don't think I have achieved the stated goal, but I am pleased about other things I have learnt or discovered, which will go towards better parenting.

- *In general*
  Looking over the work we have done together, what was most useful? What was least useful – could we have done some things differently?

  Writing things down has helped me to know what is really happening and good to be made aware of the positives. It's good to focus in on one problem so that you don't feel swamped.

- *The future*
  Now that we have finished our work together, will you try this way of doing things without me?

  I hope I can put into practice some of the improvements – there's always the fear that everything will slip back.

(Portfolio A 2000: 5.1)

The evaluation has its own processes, too, and these need not rely on question and answer routines. A few adventurous practitioners have involved people in drawing their feelings about the outcome of the work, having felt positively about their own experience of this graphic technique during the task-centred training workshops. The evaluation with Roger, a man with severe physical and learning disabilities, had to rely on accurate interpretation of his non-verbal communications and vocalisations.

Different perceptions

Even with a successful outcome and generally positive feelings about the process, some workers are surprised at the extent of people's continuing self-doubt:

> I felt much more positive about the outcome than Evelyn herself did. Evelyn lacks confidence in herself and I felt she was very hard on herself in her ratings when reviewing tasks.
>
> (Portfolio G 2000: 5.1)

> At the start of the evaluation process I made the assumption that Kelly would be very pleased with her completion of the goal. It did not occur to me that she would continue to doubt her ability. As the result of this assumption I had to think on my feet and enable Kelly to recognise her strengths and the achievements she had made while acknowledging that her thoughts were also valid. This provided me with a valuable lesson in the danger of making assumptions.
>
> (Portfolio B 2002: 5.1)

This is salutary for practitioners, a reminder that any work, task-centred or not, needs to be set in context. The work can provide a sometimes dramatic step in a new direction, but changes in the way people feel about themselves usually take repeated positive experiences.

OTHER PERSPECTIVES

The person who 'owns' the goal will have a subjective view of how far the goal has been achieved and, as we have already stated, this is the most significant perspective. However, other people's views are also relevant, especially people who are significant to the service user or carer. The view we construct of ourselves is as much a social construct as a personal one.

Practitioners often feel inhibited about involving others for fear of being seen to give power to other people in the person's life who are often seen to be relatively powerful (for example, a parent or carer, or another professional). However, to exclude these people from the evaluation is to miss an opportunity not just for this particular positive feedback, but a rehearsal for how future feedback can be given:

> Roger's uncle, who has not seen Roger for a number of years, saw a vast improvement in his social skills and contentment with his surroundings. . . . Roger's uncle said that 'however small the task appeared to others, for Roger it is a great achievement'.
>
> (Portfolio I 2003: 5.1)

> Wayne is getting on with his family much better and his mother appears to be pleased with the changes. She has been talking to Wayne about the ways that she might help him with his heroin withdrawal (alternative therapies). . . . Wayne appears to have recognised that his more reasonable behaviour in his home environment is leading to an improved relationship with his mother and the rest of the family.
>
> (Portfolio F 2003: 5.1)

In achieving a goal, or at least working towards it, people will often reference their progress in terms of how others such as family members see their efforts. These motivators should not be underestimated:

> Wayne had often felt that he was a disappointment to his mother because of his criminal and antisocial behaviour, he feels that the changes that he has made has earned him some respect in the family household.
>
> (Portfolio F 2003: 5.1)

> Sharon had discussed a little of the work with her partner but doing this wasn't something we had really talked about in sessions, and with hindsight, perhaps we should have. It would have been good for Sharon to be able to share her success more with her partner. At least if we had discussed it more, Sharon would have seen that including significant others or discussing the work with them, can be a feature of task-centred work.
>
> (Portfolio A 2000: 5.1)

It is always important to ask people's permission before seeking other perspectives on the work. Indeed, a person's task late in the work could be to seek others' views on the impact of the work. This permission is especially important when it involves other professionals. However, apart from the hope of the boost to morale which would follow an observation of positive change, this is a good opportunity to include others who may have been on the periphery of the task-centred work, but whose future involvement may be needed:

> The Housing Manager involved in Evelyn's case was both pleased and surprised at her motivation to obtain rehousing. . . . The children's social worker was also pleased that Evelyn had made so much progress as the children had been in care six months with little change in Evelyn's circumstances.
>
> (Portfolio G 2000: 5.1)

We have noted that the evaluation concerns not just the person's achievement of their goal and their experience of the work, but also the practitioner's use of the task-centred model. Other perspectives should also be sought in respect of the practitioner's work, and this is often most valuable when an observer has had the opportunity to witness the worker's direct practice with people. Informed consent must be obtained, so that this process is not seen as intrusive, but people are often keen to be able to help the development of good practice, as long as they know the purpose of any observation. One component of the task-centred portfolio is a structured observation of the learner's task-centred practice. What follows is an extract from one such evaluation:

> *What aspects of the session do you consider were the most successful?*
>
> Encouraging Wayne to reflect on the problems that he has encountered and enabling him to identify alternative tasks to help him reach his goals.
>
> *How might this session have been improved?*
>
> Laura could have spent longer checking out that Wayne fully understood next week's jobs [tasks]. He said he was clear about them but this was not checked out. His concentration appeared to be going at this point.
>
> (Portfolio F 2003: 7.2)

Of course, there are people whose lives are very isolated and for whom the practitioner's regard is pre-eminent:

> I felt it important . . . to congratulate John on his success as he had no family or friends to share his joy with. John's social worker has noticed a change in him. Not just in the achievement of his goal, but in himself. John now takes a little more pride in the things he does and has gained slightly more confidence.
>
> (Portfolio K 2002: 5.1)

See Activity 7.5

ACTIVITY 7.5: SERVICE USER AND CARER

Involving others in the work

The task-centred method encourages the involvement of other people who are directly involved in the problem or who are significant if the goal is going to be achieved.

- In what circumstances do you think other people should be involved in the review of your progress towards the goal? What can they contribute?
- In what circumstances might you not want this kind of involvement?

There is an example answer in the Appendix.

What is different for the practitioner?

As well as the question of what difference the task-centred practice has made for service users and carers, practitioners will want to ask themselves what is different about their task-centred practice from their 'regular' practice. This evaluation is important if changes are to become embedded in future work and these one or two sequences of task-centred work are not to be consigned to dusty memory. Sometimes it is possible to discover what might be different from people who have previous experience of the agency's services:

> When I asked Wayne how our work had been different from what he had experienced in the past, he recognised that we looked in depth at the outcome rather than glossing over what we had set out to do or simply forgetting about the work. In the past Wayne has talked with workers about making changes in his life but often the focus had become lost in the chaos of his lifestyle.
>
> (Portfolio F 2003: 5.2)

The service user's feedback can be very affirming for the practitioner:

> It was not until John stated that he could not have done it without me that I realised I had contributed to the success, and that my ability to reason and discuss without letting my personal perceptions get in the way, helped John to make the informed choices he needed to achieve his goal.
>
> (Portfolio K 2002: 5.2)

The portfolio offers a particularly valuable opportunity to reflect on differences between current and past practices, and ways in which the learning from the task-centred encounter is being transferred into other areas of practice. A reflective diary could serve a similar purpose.

> I intend to build into my work the principles of openness and easy access to records by offering the service user access to the recording and letter writing that has been completed by me when not in their presence between sessions.
>
> I have started to do this with service users by taking their work files into sessions and explaining the sections where information is kept, and why I need to keep such information. Although often surprised by this, I have experienced several different responses from total disinterest to a very keen interest in reading what has been written down.
>
> (Portfolio F 2003: 5.3)

In Box 7.8 we have collected fourteen quotations from practitioners' portfolios which illustrate the kinds of evaluations which people have made in respect of their experience of working together using the task-centred method (see Activity 7.6).

BOX 7.8: WHAT THEY SAID ABOUT TASK-CENTRED WORKING

1 The family was asked what they thought of this way of working. Diana said she had not had any involvement with social services before, and didn't really know what to expect. She said she didn't expect to be involved in the work, rather that we were going to tell her what was wrong. Diana said that when she contacted social services the only thing she had thought of was Mat's behaviour towards her and his stepfather and she wanted this to stop. Working in this way had given her an opportunity to understand *why* Mat behaved in this way.

(Portfolio D 2002: 5.2)

2 Using the task-centred model had helped Evelyn understand her problems more and she also gained a better understanding of why her children had been taken into care. It also gave her the means and encouragement to bring about changes in her life which would affect the outcome of the situation – if she had not paid off the arrears and made significant improvements to the condition of her house she would not have been rehoused and the children would not have been returned to her. I therefore feel that the work contributed to increasing her power. At the end of the work I felt very proud of Evelyn . . . she had worked really hard to improve her situation and this had restored in her some self-confidence and self-respect.

(Portfolio G 2000: 5)

3 From a social worker's perspective, knowing that by the end of our work together we would be evaluating the outcome enabled me to keep focused and motivated towards achieving the ultimate goals rather than getting sidetracked by the many other issues which were relevant to Wayne.

(Portfolio F 2003: 5.1)

4 It was a joint learning process and we both [worker and service user] understood more about the process at the end, than at the beginning.

(Portfolio A 2000: 5.2)

5 It enabled us both [worker and service user] to separate one piece of work from another, giving a greater chance of achievable success. Ending one piece of work before beginning another ensured we remained focused when we could easily have become side-tracked.

(Portfolio A 2000: 5.2)

6 Evelyn had been looking forward to the sessions . . . because she felt as though she wasn't being told what to do.

(Portfolio G 2000: 5.2)

7 My overall feeling at this stage [well into the Task Implementation stage] was how versatile and adaptable the task-centred model is.

(Portfolio G 2000: 4.2)

8 It wasn't until I tried the task-centred model that I realised our endings [in this unit] were not as clear as I thought they were . . . and that it is important for both client and worker to see that the ending is built into the beginning.

(Portfolio C 1995: 6)

9 In circumstances where a client denies that there is a problem at all, the task-centred method is not readily applicable. However, I think we can still take principles from it, e.g. building on client strengths to boost their confidence and reduce the fear some clients have of social work intervention.

(Portfolio A 2000: 1.4)

10 With previous evaluations [before I learned about task-centred practice], it has mainly consisted of 'How are things now?', and the service user would explain the current situation. Evaluating the task-centred intervention together with the family gave the opportunity to ask specific questions without there being right or wrong answers.

(Portfolio D 2002: 5.1)

11 The task-centred approach allowed Wayne to make a positive contribution to the work in deciding direction and prioritising the importance of certain issues in his life that he needed to deal with.

(Portfolio F 2003: 2.1)

12 [I asked Dave], 'Overall, what do you think about this way of working?'

[He said], 'It's OK, but I like to do things in my own time. We have got to know each other better and I can talk to you'. . . Dave said perhaps we could look at some of the other things, but not yet.

(Portfolio E 2000: 5.2D; 5.3)

13 The least successful [aspect at this stage of the work] was focusing Diana [the mother] on the problem being discussed; it seemed like she wanted to 'throw' another issue in at every opportunity and it was hard work to continually refocus Diana on what was being discussed.

(Portfolio D 2002: 3.1)

14 I had mixed feelings about the quotes: I found Luke's quotes helped me to understand the problems from his point of view and to appreciate the depth of his feelings about his problems. On the other hand, I felt that Luke thought I hadn't listened properly to his problem details and that I needed him to say something else so I'd understand. Once I'd explained that the quotes were useful to stop me putting my meaning on things he seemed to feel better about doing this.

(Portfolio C 1995: 2.2)

ACTIVITY 7.6: TRAINER

Using feedback to teach and develop task-centred practice

- How might you use some or all of the quotations in Box 7.8 with people who are learning to put the task-centred method into practice?

KEY POINTS

- □ It is important to review both processes and outcomes in the task-centred work.
- □ Reviewing tasks strengthens the working alliance between practitioners, users and carers.
- □ The task self-rating system can accelerate awareness of progress and change.
- □ Recording task-centred work is integral to the practice itself and involves service users and carers in the process itself.
- □ 'Flipcharting' has proved to be an effective technique.
- □ The overall evaluation of the work invites people to make a judgement about its value and worth. Others' perspectives can also be valuable.

KEY READING

Shaw, I. and Lishman, J. (eds) (1999) *Evaluation and Social Work Practice* London: Sage Publications

In addition to the key reading for Chapter 6, which is also relevant to this chapter, this book on evaluating social work practice is a useful guide: based firmly within social work the book offers a wide range of approaches, linking evaluation theory and method to application directly within practice.

CHAPTER 8

SUPPORT

OBJECTIVES

By the end of this chapter you should:

- Understand what is needed to sustain and support task-centred practice
- Know that sympathetic teams and workplaces are sources of support
- Appreciate the role of supervision in supporting task-centred practice
- Know some of the key elements needed for supervisory support
- Be able to design some 'self-training' support for task-centred practice.

SUPPORTING TASK-CENTRED PRACTICE

Teams are an important aspect of social care service delivery, and they also play a key role in the continuing support of task-centred work. There are a number of different ways that teams can interact with service users and with carers to sustain and develop this. Supervisors within teams will have a key role in support, and ideally they will work in ways which are consonant with the task-centred approach.

Overall, if practice is to be supported and improved, there must be a serious emphasis on education and on continuing professional development, and the idea of coaching is likely be central to this endeavour. The manager coach is probably the ideal for supporting task-centred work. As Greene and Grant (2003: 15) have noted:

> The coaching mindset is like the oil that lubricates the relationship between managers and their teams. It provides organizations with a process by which they can enable their employees to grow, change and adapt.

While senior staff, trainers, service users and team leaders all have important roles to play in supporting the approach, there is also work that the individual practitioner can do as self-help. While the main argument of this chapter is that it is wrong and ineffective to put the responsibility for change and development on the practitioner alone, there are nonetheless a number of things that they can and should do to provide their own support, and a number of ideas for self-learning approaches are outlined in the last section of this chapter.

RESEARCH, KNOWLEDGE AND PRACTICE

Task-centred work is based on a developmental learning model, where knowledge is created through practice. That practice is experienced, developed and analysed by researchers, practitioners, service users and carers. As outlined in Chapter 1, task-centred knowledge is based on the contributions of researchers, practitioners, service users and carers, a tripartite foundation as outlined by Janet Lewis (2002).

Support is therefore needed for each of these groups to make a good contribution to the knowledge. This needs support for both development and dissemination. Some, perhaps most, of the practitioner and service user contributions will be local, and all of them will, by definition, derive directly from and be directly relevant to practice. But for research there are substantial barriers to making good links to knowledge development. Diffusion of research information is a long-standing problem in all professions, and social work, in common with other professions, has paid particular attention to this problem in recent years with the development of models of research-based practice (Kirk and Reid 2002).

There are four stages which could be identified in the movement of research and its findings into usable knowledge. First, there needs to be relevant research undertaken, with funding for practice-based research, covering appropriate areas and undertaken in sufficient quantity. Then there is a dissemination stage, getting the information out to those who will work with it. This information itself needs to be translated into skills, practices, strategies and policies. This stage, the third, involves implementation of the research. Finally the work needs to be embedded in mainstream practice, it needs to be adopted as part of the everyday culture, knowledge and activities of practitioners. Research can therefore be seen as having the sequential stages of Information, Dissemination, Implementation and Adoption, a process that could be termed 'IDIA'. Each stage of IDIA has its own needs.

As we noted in Chapter 1, the provision of good and relevant research in social care has been a continuing struggle over the years. In the UK the output of social work research is significantly less than that of comparable applied disciplines. The funding available to universities for research in 2002–2003, for example, was £9,159 per staff member in social work, as compared with £17,685 for professions allied to medicine, and £20,409 for community-based clinical subjects (Fisher and Marsh 2003). Only nursing has a comparably low figure, at £9,717, but even here the growth in funding year on year is outstripping social work (86 per cent as compared with 21 per cent growth). There is a serious lack of UK research that derives from, and whose discipline base is within, social work.

Dissemination of research has a more positive history within social work in the UK. The production may be limited, but there have been numerous projects to make this material available to the practice and policy community, and more recently to service users and carers. Of particular significance may be the establishment, in 2001, of the Social Care

Institute for Excellence with a specific remit to provide electronic dissemination and to help make research materials available and useful. They can draw on good previous experience, such as that outlined in Box 8.1.

BOX 8.1: INFORMATION PRACTICE

A five-year action research project in the late 1970s, Project INISS (Information Needs In Social Services), showed that dissemination of research was vital, and that effort put into dissemination work could have substantial positive gains (Streatfield and Wilson 1980).

The project outlined an agenda which has been developed since the early 1980s:

- brief information sheets on research relevant to current policy concerns
- quick access to research abstracts to help with case decisions
- staff in specialist posts to build an organisation's knowledge of key research
- the need to cite and link research directly within procedure manuals and briefing documents.

With the development of the World Wide Web the dissemination activities have become more and more achievable. Task-centred literature is increasingly available on the desktop of a practitioner.

With task-centred work the next stage of the IDIA cycle, making sure that implementation ideas are built from the research, is also in good shape because the implementation of research-based ideas is at the core of practice. The research that is cited in this book as specifically task centred has come from practice problems, been developed in a practice setting, and has practice implications built in.

But the fourth stage of the cycle, the adoption of such research into everyday practice, looks as problematic as the first. Task-centred research can provide good implementation ideas for the training programme, but helping staff to move from this training programme to mainstream practice is hard. Sustaining task-centred practice as a day-to-day working model is difficult. It is this sustaining work that is the focus of the remaining sections of this chapter.

THE PROFESSIONAL AGENCY AS A LEARNING ORGANISATION

Task-centred practice involves the judicious use of three sources of knowledge: that from research; that from practice experience; and that from the views of service users and carers. In a social work agency it will usually involve setting this knowledge in the context of specific policies, and it will often involve some aspect of the law. Balancing up these different sources is far from easy. Doing so in a stressful situation, where there are often important consequences for the lives of individuals, is particularly difficult.

To support this complex activity agencies need to promote the thoughtfulness of their staff, and provide them with an environment in which that thinking can draw upon the best current knowledge. An immediate response to these issues would be to say that agencies need good training programmes to keep staff up to date, and good information materials for them to use. While both of these elements are important they are not likely to be sufficient for the best support of task-centred practice. Learning needs to continue beyond training, and information materials need to make the most of difficult-to-capture ideas which are based in, for example, practice experience and service user preferences. How can an organisation promote learning, and how can it build in these ideas?

The most promising avenue for an organisation to follow, and one which has had management development work (Iles and Sutherland 2001), is to develop itself as a learning organisation.

Learning organisations are one step on from effective, efficient and ethical organisations. They need these three traits in order to be competent at their current tasks, just like any good organisation. But they are also capable of continuing to be good at their job in the context of changing demands on them and of changing opportunities for them. The learning organisation should be good at its work now and also in a few years time when there are new laws and new services. Learning organisations respond positively to changes in their environment, and to new developments in practice. In both these areas there are parallels with task-centred practice, which adjusts to the views and wishes of service users (and law and policy-makers), and consciously seeks to enhance its practice by a developmental model (see Box 8.2).

Learning organisations should provide the overall support that task-centred practice needs, a climate and culture of learning within the whole organisation (Pedler and Aspinwall 1998).

The size of the organisational unit that can be the learning organisation may well vary. For many task-centred practitioners it will be their team that is the most important 'organisation' for their support. If the team can express the learning, changing, developing elements of the learning organisation then that will be an important support at the organisational level for them. Helping smaller units support learning organisation behaviour is also likely to be easier, and it may well be that staff who work in smaller agencies, most commonly found in the voluntary, private and not-for-profit sector, will have the greatest success in promoting learning organisation work (see Activity 8.1).

ACTIVITY 8.1: MANAGER

What would an agency that has developed itself as a learning organisation look like?

Consider the organisation that you manage, and reflect on the following questions:

- Are there systems for reviewing the effectiveness of policy change and associated training?
- Does the policy and budget for training allow for a flexible development of learning, involving, for example, service users in change work?
- Are staff at all levels encouraged to play a role in development and change?
- Do teams allocate time for development, and do workload systems, as well as job descriptions, give recognition to development work?

There is an example answer in the Appendix.

BOX 8.2: THE LEARNING ORGANISATION

Here is a succinct definition of the key elements of a learning organisation.

Structure

Learning organisations have managerial hierarchies that enhance opportunities for employee, carer and service user involvement in the organisation. All are empowered to make relevant decisions. Structures support teamwork and strong lateral relations (not just vertical). Networking is enabled across organisational and hierarchical boundaries both internally and externally

Organisational culture

Learning organisations have strong cultures that promote openness, creativity and experimentation among members. They encourage members to acquire, process and share information, nurture innovation and provide the freedom to try new things, to risk failure and to learn from mistakes.

Information systems

Learning organisations require information systems that improve and support practice and that move beyond that used in traditional organisations where information is generally used for control purposes. 'Transformational change' requires more sophisticated information systems that facilitate rapid acquisition, processing and sharing of rich, complex information that enables effective knowledge management.

Human resource practices

People are recognised as the creators and users of organisational learning. Accordingly, human resource management focuses on provision and support of individual learning. Appraisal and reward systems are concerned to measure long-term performance and to promote the acquisition and sharing of new skills and knowledge.

Leadership

Like most interventions aimed at securing significant organisational improvement, organisational learning depends heavily on effective leadership. Leaders model the openness, risk taking and reflection necessary for learning and communicate a compelling vision of the learning organisation, providing empathy, support and personal advocacy needed to lead others towards it. They ensure that organisations and work groups have the capacity to learn, change and develop.

(Based on Iles and Sutherland 2001: 65)

Ideally the learning organisation will have staff at all levels, actively engaged with service users and carers, promoting and sustaining learning. This will provide an excellent overall environment for task-centred practice.

A DEVELOPMENTAL WORKPLACE

All practitioners will engage with people outside of their team, and outside of the formal line hierarchy within their organisation, because of the requirements of their practice. They will need to work with people in specialist posts, with people in different service sections, with colleagues in other similar teams, and so on. Equally they will work with a wide variety of people outside of their organisation. This will include, for example, different professional groups, service user advocates, colleagues in other similar organisations, and so on. These contacts, based on the needs of their work, will normally arise because of attempts to solve particular problems in the work, or because of some form of pre-existing joint working. 'Practice' will, by definition, be central to these relationships.

These relationships, external to the team, will be part of the development of practice, with varying levels of success, for specific situations. Sometimes, perhaps normally, they will be supportive for the practitioner. They are part of continuing learning, and part of a continuing process of development of practice. If they are, or mostly are, helpful in this way they will form part of a wider developmental workplace for the practitioner.

But just how supportive such activities are likely to be, and just how developmental the workplace, will be driven by factors that are beyond the practitioner's control. It may be that these workplace relationships are strongly biased to particular outside groups, excluding excellent sources of learning. Luck will enter into the process, and some task-centred workers will not find much support for task-centred principles, nor much knowledge of task-centred work. Since the mid-1990s there has been growing interest in more deliberate development of a supportive workplace to run alongside the service-driven contacts. This can provide allies within and without the organisation who can help to support and develop task-centred practice.

The idea of pulling together a community that shares a common practice interest, to utilise the skills and experiences of the group to develop that practice, has been shown to be both effective and well liked. These 'communities of practice' are 'groups of people who share a concern, a set of problems, or a passion about a topic, and who deepen their knowledge and expertise in this area by interacting on an ongoing basis' (Wenger *et al.* 2002: 4). The results of their work in private and public sector settings have been impressive, not least in the sense that they are the 'social fabric' of learning organisations (Wenger 1998: 253).

Communities of practice can provide many of the elements of support that we have been discussing so far. They can provide ways in which information is made accessible and pooled, for example by running some form of shared system for finding and storing relevant literature. They can provide support by sharing professional experience. Service user and carer members can bring their knowledge to the community. They might provide social support by meeting, they might provide motivational support by celebrating success, and of course in the age of the internet they can be, in varying degree, virtual, thereby reducing the overheads of travel and aiding accessibility.

Communities of practice can provide access to and exchange of ideas, and they can develop practice in a variety of ways (see Box 8.3). But they are not just a project group, or a social support mechanism, although there will be elements of both. They come together for more than a one-off project, and they act as a means of identification with practice that moves well beyond social support. They provide the possibility for everyone to be a leader in the development of the shared practice. While there will be nominated convenors, and possibly a librarian and a secretary, the community is a shared enterprise based around mutual norms. It is not part of a given structure of an organisation, and does not rely on leaders who lead and followers who follow. All may lead, in different ways and at different times (Drath and Palus 1994). The links with some of the underlying partnership and development principles of task-centred practice are strong.

BOX 8.3: COMMUNITIES OF PRACTICE

Seven principles for developing a community of practice.

1 *Design for evolution*
Allow for change and development within the community and in terms of its objectives and processes.
2 *Open a dialogue between inside and outside perspectives*
Make sure there is communication between those inside the community and those outside it, especially about the community's potential achievements.
3 *Invite different levels of participation*
Allow different members of the community to engage in the way they want, with different levels of involvement at different times.
4 *Develop both public and private community spaces*
Informal and formal community events are both important to success.
5 *Focus on value*
Be explicit about the value being delivered by the community. Work hard to express this in ways that community members and others can understand, in terms of examples of contribution to specific policies, organisational aims and efficiency goals.
6 *Combine familiarity and excitement*
People like the familiar, it helps them feel comfortable and able to contribute, but there also needs to be excitement to challenge thinking and to maintain interest over the longer term.
7 *Create a rhythm for the community*
Some regular pattern to community events is good for making sure that members stay engaged and do not drift away.

(Based on Wenger *et al.* 2002: 49–64)

Communities of practice also provide an opportunity for the continuing support which is needed as part of any training development (Newton and Marsh 1993) and a form of coaching and mentoring (Parsloe and Wray 2000) that is relatively egalitarian and based directly on practice skills. Training could help to support the communities, and the idea of communities of practice has informed the training suggestions made in this book (see Activity 8.2).

ACTIVITY 8.2: TRAINER

How could training help to support 'a community of practice'?

Read the seven principles of developing a community of practice in Box 8.3 again. How could training help support these principles? What would a training programme look like that supported these principles?

THE TEAM

Alongside communities of practice the existing work team could be developed to provide both support and development for task-centred practice. Some focus on the team is undoubtedly important even if a community of practice can be developed. Team members are in contact daily, and could provide an important source of encouragement for task-centred principles.

The team can also play a more destructive role. Staff returning from post-qualifying training, for example, have sometimes found that their new knowledge and skills are not valued by their team mates, and indeed they may find that they are actively opposed (Rushton and Martyn 1990). If individual training is undertaken, then building in some form of 're-entry' work is likely to be important, a point we will return to later.

The manner of possible team support will be different from team to team, in part dependent on personality, history, organisational culture, and so on. However, it will notably depend on the way that the team itself works together. All teams will share a common objective or objectives, and all will have some clear sense of membership, but beyond this there is a spectrum with different amounts of shared skills and of close face-to-face partnership work. A useful analogy for the spectrum is to consider the nature of sporting teams (Payne and Scott 1982).

The athletics team has groups of people in similar sports, but individuals are typically relatively independent within their group, and it is unusual to be able to interchange with another group. Fitness may be common to team members, but skills are usually very different from sport to sport. Team members can provide support to one to another, but between sport groups they can provide very little feedback, and even within one sport group detailed feedback is needed from a coach rather than fellow team member. The athletics 'team' is in reality more of a close network. Individuals will seek support from fellow sport members, and from the whole team to some degree, but they will develop via personal coaching on their own track.

The football team, on the other hand, has much more of a common base to the skills of its players, and within limits a good degree of interchangeability. Members need to work together in a co-ordinated way, and feedback between members is possible and important to team development. Individuals will look to bring colleagues firmly along with them, to provide feedback on their work as it progresses, to share skills and ideas, and the coach will emphasise these factors.

On the spectrum from the athletics to the football team, there may be a midway point occupied by tennis. Here success depends on winning a series of matches, and doubles play requires close co-ordination between players. There is a good degree of interchangeability within singles play, but many singles players are not good doubles players (or do not want to dilute their singles skills in the different type of game), and doubles partners build up a close knowledge of each other's play that is not amenable to quick substitution of another player. Individuals will seek some feedback from other players, and if in doubles will need very close shared work, with coaches encouraging different mixes of team and individual development throughout.

What sort of team you are part of will therefore affect the type and quality of support and feedback you can expect (see Activity 8.3). Residential care teams will probably be most like football teams, and large multidisciplinary teams most like athletic teams.

ACTIVITY 8.3: PRACTITIONER

What kind of support and feedback should the experienced practitioner seek in their team?

- Consider who you should look to for *support*, and who you should look to for *feedback* in your team.
- Given your team, which team members do you think will be most appropriate for mutual support of your work?
- Does your type of team provide an opportunity for close co-ordinated working between individuals? If so, will this provide good feedback for your work, and how might this be encouraged?

SERVICE USERS

This chapter began by emphasising again the tripartite nature of knowledge in social care. The views of service users and carers sit alongside professional expertise and research in providing the foundation for practice. Task-centred work emphasises this in the core of its approach when considering mandates and agreements for practice, and in the development of tasks to enact them. It also requires user and carer views to be built into developmental work in terms of feedback on practice both during and at the end of periods of service, where user and carer comments should highlight areas that professionals could improve as well as areas that seem to succeed.

There is a wider developmental role for service users and carers who can, and if possible should, play a role in supporting task-centred work as a means of effective partnership practice for social care. Beyond the individual experience of service there could be contributions to the ways that teams support task-centred practice, for example by user groups working with a team to provide a summary of good and poor practice as they see it and then seeing how this stands up to the principles of task-centred work. A number of innovative routes to engage more closely with service users and carers could be followed; for example, could there be the social care equivalent of a school parents' evening, but where the reports on performance were gathered from service users and carers and presented to professionals?

Service users and carers have a right to expect the most efficient, effective and ethical service that is realistically possible, and their support of task-centred work will be an important element in providing this (see Activity 8.4).

ACTIVITY 8.4: SERVICE USER AND CARER

What would you expect from a task-centered worker?

Service users and carers might want to ask, as part of their analysis of the working partnership with social workers, what the skills, knowledge and experience are of the workers they are seeing. As a service user or carer, what answers would you expect from a task-centred worker?

There is an example answer in the Appendix.

THE SUPERVISOR

Supervision has a central role in supporting good practice. It can, for example, provide a means of maintaining key practice principles, help good analysis in emotional situations and aid good decision making. It is a skilled activity and it merits serious attention.

There is some evidence that supervision may be struggling to play its important role to the full. In a UK-wide study of qualified social workers in their first year of practice, around one-fifth reported that they had no supervision in their first year (Marsh and Triseliotis 1996: 151). The supervision that is carried out may emphasise one part of the task to the exclusion of others, for example focusing predominantly on resources (Richards *et al.* 1990) and being fuzzily protective of staff (Pithouse 1998). The worries that have been expressed for many years about supervision losing a key educational role (Clare 1988) have some grounds in the literature, and it is this educational role that is the predominant concern of this chapter. Providing this role may be quite a challenge for supervisors, but good support for task-centred work depends on them rising to it.

The areas of support that have already been discussed will all benefit from a supervisor's attention. At a broad policy level there needs to be a willingness to promote the ideas and practices underpinning learning organisations, and there is a range of indirect support for task-centred practice which could be provided by promoting communities of practice, team feedback, and user and carer involvement. Specifically it will be helpful for the process of development of task-centred work to be incorporated directly into the supervision agenda. This could involve establishing the commitment of team members to supporting training and development time, and it will certainly involve paying attention to the re-entry from training that was described as a problem earlier. Staff developing new skills need to know that their supervisors will work to make sure that these skills are used, and that colleagues support each other in the process of change. To do this involves making sure that underlying principles of task-centred work are shared, or at least tolerated.

If supervisors are going to support this process, and to support staff directly in supervision, then they too must share the underlying principles of the work. If they do not then, at best, there will be little continuing development of the practice, and at worst it may end completely.

Task-centred supervision needs to be built with supervisors who are sympathetic to the principles of knowledge development, and of partnership, that underpin task-centred practice. A graphic example of the effects of the lack of such sympathy was provided in a task-centred developmental project in the late 1980s which had to be abandoned because:

> workers who liked the model told [the researcher] that they wished their supervisors would work with them the way they were expected to work with clients. Their attempts to use the model increased their discomfort with supervision. This lack of consonance between direct-practice models and supervision and management models confused workers and confounded their ability to use the model.
>
> (Bricker-Jenkins 1990: 13)

An effective practice system needs to be explicit in its values, internally consistent and reinforcing. Supervisors are likely to be the key to making this happen. They will be able to do so without detailed knowledge of all aspects of task-centred work, and without substantial experience of the model, although both may be advantageous if possible. They need to be committed to basic principles, and to understand enough about the broad techniques of practice, so that they can analyse work that is presented and contrast it with principles and techniques that are 'good practice' in task-centred work.

An analogy from the academic world may help to support this point. A supervisor of a postgraduate student undertaking a research dissertation will usually begin knowing more than the student about the area under study. By the end of the student's work the supervisor will almost certainly be learning from the student. But throughout the work supervisors will need to find ways to encourage best practice in research, for example the upholding of good ethical standards, and the use of appropriate research methods.

This approach to supervision, enabling people to learn and change, rather than engaging in direct teaching or instruction, has many parallels with coaching. Bearing in mind that social work supervision will inevitably spend a good deal of time on the allocation and management of resources, it is important that task-centred supervisors make sure they offer some genuine coaching, and make sure that they emphasise 'managing as a coach' (Parsloe and Wray 2000: 56).

Supervisors will need to help people learn how to learn, and to provide good feedback on ideas and on skills, sometimes by observation. There are now good texts on these areas (Le Riche and Tanner 1998; Parsloe and Wray 2000) and they should undoubtedly be part of the supervisor's key reading.

There is of course a difference between supervision of task-centred practice, and task-centred supervision, where the latter is using task-centred principles and practice directly within supervision, rather than being informed by them to support the practice of a worker (see Activity 8.5). Recent developments in task-centred work have been along these directions (Caspi and Reid 2002) but this is beyond the scope of this book.

ACTIVITY 8.5: SUPERVISOR

What would supervision to support task-centred work look like?

Prepare yourself for a supervision session by making sure that you

- know that you and your supervisee will jointly understand the aims of the coming supervision session, for example by a brief recap of an existing supervision agreement, or by explicit agreement for the session
- have a sense of the problems that may be brought to the session, so that you can plan time to make sure decisions are genuinely shared

- have a mental or real note of colleagues who you think may be supportive of the task-centred work in the team or elsewhere
- plan to cover all the different stages of task-centred work over the course of a number of sessions, and not get diverted all the time to one particular stage. Box 8.4 may help as a checklist to do this.

BOX 8.4: AN AIDE-MEMOIRE FOR SUPERVISORS: KEY ELEMENTS AND BASIC PRINCIPLES OF TASK-CENTRED WORK

Mandate

- Is it clear who is defining the problem?
- What would you do *if* the service user said, 'I don't want to see you'?
- Why are you involved?
- Is the mandate clear for all who are contracting for the work?

Problem

- Are service user and carer quotes being used?
- Is there a reasonable sense of headline, story and priority as in the newspaper metaphor?
- Are service user and carer strengths and past achievements clear enough?
- Is any legally imposed problem clearly expressed?

Goals

- Are they SMART?
- Is the causal link between goal and problem reasonably understood?
- Are goals ethically sound, and reasonably in the control of the service users and carers?

Time limit

- Is there one?!

Tasks

- Are tasks well understood, and created in some form of partnership?
- Has the Task Planning and Implementation Sequence been used?
- How has task development and review contributed to learning?

Review

- Is a review of progress built into all the practice, but not overwhelmingly?

There can be times when helping people to learn is difficult because of the wealth of areas to be covered. It is easy as learner or coach to be overwhelmed. Looking at key elements of the task-centred approach and the underlying principles within them may be one way to avoid this problem.

SELF-POWERED SUPPORT

Examination of the support needed to promote task-centred practice has involved looking at the nature of the knowledge required, the nature of the organisation and groups that will help, and how others, such as supervisors and service users and carers, can help. But what about the individual? How can individuals help to support themselves?

Developing and supporting any complex, difficult activity, like task-centred practice, involves both motivation and focused attention on skill development. Going to the gym is something many people want to do, but 'forcing yourself' to do it after a day's work, on a cold wet night, is usually far from easy. Motivation is required to get us going, and then we have to find ways to concentrate on the skill development. That concentration, whether on the details of the gym stretching exercise, or on the correct way to use the rowing machine, must also be productive. Too much concentration and we can sometimes feel paralysed by the difficulty of the task, and having won the motivation battle we lose heart at this stage, because it is 'all too difficult'.

Doing one's best to provide self-support to tackle these two issues involves a degree of self-reflection, and this will be helpful in learning, and may also address some of the issues we have covered in Chapter 5. Motivation is going to reflect a particular combination of personality, job, stage of career, and perhaps other factors that will be unique for each individual. The key issue for self-support is to engage, as honestly and accurately as possible, in analysis of this for your circumstances. There is no magic motivation potion available for all, but there is likely to be one, albeit sometimes rather dilute, that works pretty well for you – especially true as you have read this far in this book (see Activity 8.6).

ACTIVITY 8.6: LEARNER

Self-support: sustaining motivation

Make a list of the different factors that would motivate you to develop your work on task-centred practice.

These could include, for example:

- the views that service users and carers have of your work
- a contribution to your CV that might aid your career
- the intellectual challenges of continuing to learn task-centred practice
- a work partnership that you would like to develop, and so on.

Spend a few minutes on this, attempt to provide as wide a range as possible.
Then rank the factors in priority order, and for the top ones provide a note as to how you might reinforce the process. An example from each of those above could be:

- make a file of 'good news' from service user feedback
- update your CV with concrete examples
- take stock of what you have learnt in a reflective notebook
- agree with a colleague to work this way, and so on.

If reasonable attempts are made to make sure that motivation is kept as high as possible, how can one ensure that development is not stopped by the sheer difficulty of trying to do it all right in circumstances that nearly always seem to conspire against you. The paralysis referred to earlier will set in if concentration is too high. It will stop you building your skills stage by stage, because too much thought on the myriad things that you should do right to achieve the perfect Task Planning and Implementation Sequence, will stop you getting that sequence right. In the coaching world this is a well-known effect (Gallwey 1986), with advice that you should work on your inner game, and make sure that you are not overwhelmed by your own self-criticism or too many conflicting points from experts.

The solution in the task-centred approach is to go back to the basic principles, which will also have the effect of reminding you why you are working in this way and aid motivation. Going back to these basic principles allows you to develop at your own speed, and probably relaxes you, which should then allow skills to develop in ways that were hindered by over-concentration. Observe yourself, without too much blame, against the yardstick of these principles, and development should restart. Letting yourself learn is the best form of support you can have (see Activity 8.7).

ACTIVITY 8.7: ALL

Developing 'inner task-centredness'

Whatever your particular part in a recent social work encounter, measure your experience of that encounter against the principles below. Visualise what you could have done differently to make the 'fit' with the principles better. Accept that what was done was done – you are not looking to criticise yourself or others. You are just trying to develop a vision of how it could be better next time.

- A direct expression of the views of the people involved: to form a clear mandate for the work, relevant to the culture and heritage of the service user or carer, and set alongside any mandate derived from the law.
- Clear, agreed, relevant and achievable goals: the key to working across difference, and providing direction, motivation and development of skills and strengths.
- Tasks as drivers for change: they should be showing progress, building on skills, developing skills, or revealing a lack of skills or resources that will be covered by future tasks.
- Reviewing progress: review in a mutually agreeable fashion with unambiguous indicators of progress is necessary but not sufficient for change to be long lasting.

KEY POINTS

- ☐ Research into practice involves attention to four areas: the information itself, dissemination of it, implementation of it in practice, and its adoption into the mainstream.
- ☐ A learning organisation is the ideal setting for task-centred work because of the climate of development and learning that is part of this approach.
- ☐ Communities of practice would provide a good way for task-centred work to develop via the shared experience of those directly engaging in the practice itself.
- ☐ Teams can be supportive, but analysing the type of team you are in, and the ways it operates, will be important to maximising that support.
- ☐ Supervision can be a key support for task-centred practice, especially if the focus is on helping people learn how to learn, and providing good feedback on staff ideas and skills.
- ☐ Providing 'self-powered' support will be important for task-centred practitioners, and both motivation and concentration will need to be analysed to provide this successfully.

KEY READING

Parsloe, E. and Wray, M. (2000) *Coaching and Mentoring* London: Kogan Page

This covers the theory and practice of coaching and mentoring with many practical exercises and examples.

Pedler, M. and Aspinwall, K. (1998) *A Concise Guide to the Learning Organization* London: Lemos & Crane

This provides a concise summary of the key issues concerning learning organisations.

CHAPTER 9

REDEVELOP

OBJECTIVES

By the end of this chapter you should:

- Recognise the importance of developing social work practice
- Have considered whether it matters that 'task-centred work' *is* task-centred
- Recognise the role of individuals, groups and structures in the development of social work practice
- Know how task-centred practice fits with current issues in social work practice
- Understand how task-centred practice could benefit future practice.

CONTINUING TO DEVELOP TASK-CENTRED PRACTICE

We have argued throughout this book that service users and carers will receive the best service only if there is sustained and concentrated attention paid to the development and support of direct social work practice. The knowledge for this practice should be explicitly and clearly based on three pillars: the evidence from research, practice wisdom and the experiences and wishes of service users and carers. The mix of this knowledge will vary from situation to situation, from person to person, and from setting to setting. Social work practice needs to be explicit and serious about these three contributions, and to find practical ways of developing this knowledge. We have shown how task-centred practice is explicit, serious and practical in connection with these three pillars. But we have also shown that moving from this knowledge, and from the task-centred model, to the delivery of these ideas is far from simple. Moving from 'knowing' to 'doing' in social work, is at the heart of task-centred practice. This process is complex and requires good models of learning, and of personal, team and agency support and development. It requires understanding the learning that is needed for the journey from knowing to doing in the real world of social work.

Task-centred practice requires sustained development effort. This work fits well with ideas of 'best practice' in connection with learning organisations and with communities of practice (as we outlined in Chapter 8). New task-centred practitioners need good learning models to begin the work, and then sustained use of learning to move it into mainstream practice. Supervision of this practice must provide for proper accountability. The ability of an organisation and its practitioners to respond well to the people it serves will need to be seriously examined and resourced. There are good models to help with this examination and we have outlined them in this book. Providing good task-centred practice fits excellently with best practice in partnership work with service user and carers, in providing accountability and in promoting flexible and responsive social services. It fits very well with the continuing promotion of a wider citizen participation agenda, even if it does not directly address it (Payne 1997). It makes no claims to do so. Work must take place both on the wider agenda, and on the direct practice element of social work. It is the latter that has been so ignored and it is time to take it seriously again. It is time to continue the development of task-centred practice because it can do so much, in so many practical ways, to enhance the lives of service users and carers.

Focusing on the knowledge for, and the methods of, direct practice is an increasingly urgent need, not least because of the administrative and rule-bound surrogate which is displacing professional practice in social work. In a national study of social workers in training and their first year of work (Marsh and Triseliotis 1996), it was found that practitioners had great difficulty in receiving support for professional analysis, for professional practice, but they were faced with a requirement to follow increasingly prescriptive bureaucratic rules. Providing guidelines for practice is an excellent idea (providing they are clearly based on the three pillars we outlined above, and they are firmly located in the real world of social work), but providing a detailed manual of what you do when will result in an administrative service, not a professional one. For some circumstances, perhaps most, this may work well, but social work has been charged with the task of working with people in complex situations, often unable or unwilling to meet societal norms: following rule 3a, b, c and then 4a, b, c is an inadequate response for people who need social workers. It is of course part of the wider managerialist agenda in the late twentieth and early twenty-first centuries (see for example Clarke *et al.* 2000), but it is vital, if we are to provide high quality social work for people, that we maintain proper professional accountability (for example, via registration of social workers) and also proper professional work. Again the message is clear, we must focus on and develop professional practice, and task-centred work provides an excellent opportunity for us to do just that.

We are arguing for the development of knowledge for practice, and the ability to move that knowledge into practice action. Developing the knowledge will be a challenge in the context of its neglect. Research is rarely conducted by practitioners, and researchers are rarely engaged directly in practice. Compare the situation in health, where nearly all reasonably experienced practitioners engage in some way with research. In social work, practice is isolated on so many sides. Team leaders' practice is often restricted to attendance at reviews, accompanying staff on a difficult visit, or covering for sickness. Compare the situation in schools, where nearly all teaching staff in a school do some teaching, and rewards are high for those who stay in practice.

Building on the positive developments in social work, around for example registration of social workers, the investments made in social work basic education, and the growing recognition of the need for continuing professional development, will be difficult in the context of the extraordinarily low profile of practice. Task-centred work forms an excellent vehicle to build on those positive developments and to provide the practice base that is so important to high quality services.

HOW DO WE KNOW IT *IS* 'TASK-CENTRED' – AND DOES IT MATTER?

The frequency with which the term 'task-centred' is used in the portfolios written by social work students would suggest it is the clear method of choice in social work practice. We reviewed 25 student portfolios taken at random from a total of 41. We read the section about social work methods used during the placement, and found that 17 of the 25 portfolios (68 per cent) referred to task-centred practice, with 40 mentions of 'task-centred' in total. Task-centred work was noted more than twice as often as the next method, *crisis intervention*, which figured in 8 portfolios. Using the term 'method' loosely, other methods which were noted in 4 or more portfolios were: *counselling* (7), *advocacy and empowerment* (7), *groupwork* (6), *cognitive work* (5) and *family therapy* (4). We should note that the placement occurred before any class-based teaching of task-centred practice, so there was no sensitisation to the method prior to the placement learning.

However, task-centred was more likely to be mentioned than described or appraised. Often it was unclear how or whether task-centred was put into practice (or indeed any of the other methods), or what kind of tuition on practice methods students experienced during the placement. 'Method' was loosely interpreted to include social work principles, programmes, techniques, skills and theories. This is illustrated by the different words which followed *task-centred:*

task-centred *approach*	12 mentions in 10 portfolios
task-centred *(social) work*	9 mentions in 8 portfolios
task-centred *(practice) method*	13 mentions in 6 portfolios
task-centred *way*	3 mentions in 2 portfolios
task-centred *model*	2 mentions in 1 portfolio
task-centred *framework*	1 mention in 1 portfolio

On the basis of these findings, can we say that two out of three students are learning and practising task-centred social work?

Unfortunately, there are so many misconceptions about task-centred work that we must question whether it is really as prevalent as these portfolios suggest. For example, there is a common view that task-centred work is 'just' about doing practical things: tackling accommodation difficulties, sorting out bills and the like. For example, one practice teacher wrote:

> The student engaged this young woman in Crisis Intervention (following admission to Accident and Emergency through massive overdoses of insulin), Counselling (to assess the situation), Psychotherapy, both sexual and cogni-

> tive (to seek disclosures of earlier childhood sexual abuse to instil feelings of self-worth) and task-centred approaches (*to enable the client to realise some of her immediate income maintenance and accommodation problems*).
>
> (our emphasis)

True, it *is* a practical way of working, and 'just' helping with material problems is usually a complex job and one which is greatly appreciated. However, it is a mistake to assume that helping somebody with a practical problem is, in itself, an example of task-centred practice; conversely, task-centred work is not confined to dealing with material difficulties, as is apparent throughout this book.

Since task-centred practice is so frequently seen as synonymous with practical work, it is often wrongly contrasted with 'relationship work'. Shemmings (1991: 93) writes, 'Take, for example, methods which emphasize the importance of the quality of the relationship between worker and user *in contrast to* those stressing the delineation of tasks and objectives' (our emphasis). Since relationship work is frequently perceived as superior to practical work, task-centred practice falls prey to a certain professional snobbery. 'Life, and therefore social work, is infinitely more complex and messy – and therefore exciting – than these (contract-based and task-centred) methods often redolent of the language of management, usually permit' (Shemmings 1991: 63). Sadly, we do not discover what exciting methods were used.

On the basis of the portfolios we read, some practitioners seemed to view a social work method, any method, as something approaching an instrument of torture, with visions of service users and carers constrained and squeezed into a practice method by heartless, method-crazy practitioners. Suspicion of the idea of a practice method was widespread. However, we found no evidence of concern that people could fall victim to the *absence* of a practice method, nor was there any description of how students learned the difficult art of discrimination in their use of different practice methods. Genuine curiosity about developing skill in any particular method was rare, and in a number of cases the message was hostile, favouring some undefined eclecticism. It is unlikely that students can become familiar with enough practice methods to refine them into eclectic practice.

There is no doubt that the term 'task-centred' misleads. The word 'task' is associated with chore, duty, labour, hard task master. It can conjure unrelenting steadfastness, inflexibility, telling people what to do, tasks being assigned by one person for another to complete. Task wrongly implies physical activity, so it seems to exclude people who are not capable of moving or doing and tends to suggest that the social worker needs to get on with it all. We can see how the combination of these misconceptions places task-centred as a quick-fix technique for sorting out practical difficulties, leaving other methods to work with the real, deeper, longer-lasting problems with relationships.

As will be very clear to the reader by this point, task-centred social work is, first and foremost, a way of working with people which emphasises partnership. The meaning of *partnership* is in danger of being devalued through overuse, but we see it as a careful negotiation between people to agree what should be done and how it can be done. Part of this negotiation is an openness about how different people see the situation, about the different power and status in the relationship (between all the parties involved – workers, users and carers), and a commitment to balancing that power as far as practical and desirable.

Avoiding the question of practice method, or masquerading ignorance as eclecticism, is no answer to the issue of how people can have more control over the work, if they want it. Using the tag 'task-centred' as a catch-all for a kind of general practice which is vaguely related to practical problems is dishonest.

Does it matter whether students are practising the real thing when they write about it in their portfolios? Well, we can begin to redevelop something only when we are confident of what it is that has been developed. In terms of working in partnership, for example, we need to know whether a social work method is likely to increase the opportunities for partnership over the absence of any method, and we need to know which methods are likely to increase it more than others. Developing a partnership is not a haphazard process and we need to know which elements of an encounter, task-centred or not, have been most successful in promoting the partnership. In the task-centred method we have a systematic approach which helps us to transfer learning from one encounter to another, which is at the heart of redeveloping practice.

AN AGENDA FOR REDEVELOPMENT

Service users and carers need the ideas in this book to be taken forward, and they will have an important role in doing this, via, we hope, their involvement in a wide range of agency developments, and also of course via their role in the task-centred process itself. Practitioners, supervisors and managers need to take the ideas forward, and will benefit not only from providing a better service, but also from doing so in a setting where the heart of their work is highly valued and where the learning required to do it is actively promoted. Trainers will benefit from the ideas via more relevant training, and via seeing that the fruits of training are sustained beyond the course, and those responsible for the structures that monitor and guide social work will also benefit when the practice that is clearly at the centre of their concerns also has a real and evident theoretical, skills and knowledge base.

What might change for individuals, for groups and for structures if the development of task-centred practice was taken seriously over the coming years? How will we know if we are going down this route? We offer some ideas for key indicators to show it is happening in Box 9.1.

BOX 9.1: SOME KEY INDICATORS THAT TASK-CENTRED DEVELOPMENT IS OCCURRING

Individuals as supervisors or trainers

- *Supervision*: a movement from 'case of the day' to a more structured learning model of supervision, with a particular focus on the mandate for work and achieving agreed goals.
- *Training*: a much closer involvement with practice, with more involvement of service users and carers in training, and follow-up of training work.

Social work stakeholder groups

- *Social work teams*: a focus on sharing ideas around tasks, with more joint working based on more explicit service goals, and a shared team approach to knowledge development and service user and carer involvement.
- *Agencies*: the needs of practice as one of the key principles for the organisation of the agency, for example a practitioner as part of all development groups, a recognition of the need to keep staff in practice, with length in practice clearly valued, and practice consultant posts common.
- *Service users and carers*: direct engagement with designing feedback and evaluation models, helping with language and clarity, engaged in training, logging task ideas, and active participants in knowledge and service development.
- *The profession*: senior practitioners, alongside or in place of managers at top-level discussions and in top-level posts, a growing inter-professional agenda because social work and its role is more understandable to others, new professional journals with practitioners writing and researching for them.
- *Social work academy*: academics with substantial practice skills, more interchange of academy and field, the most difficult work in social work being dealt with by the most senior staff, so professors or consultants working in the most complex areas of practice.

Structures for social work

- *Registration*: codes of practice that include the requirement to develop practice and provide knowledge for practice, and continuing professional development that is clearly linked to three pillars of practice knowledge.
- *Guidance*: assessment frameworks that are guidelines and not detailed manuals, based on the idea that the assessment was provided primarily to aid the service user and carer in their planning.
- *Social work education*: providing a slimmed-down methods range with common principles (for example the mandate for practice running through all sections of the course) but much greater emphasis on application, with practice development at the heart of courses and linked to practice learning sites providing both student training and knowledge development.

TASK-CENTRED PRACTICE'S POTENTIAL

There are many current themes in social work which resonate with task-centred practice. First and foremost is the increasing desire, requirement and opportunity for service users and carers to have a meaningful voice, not just in their own contact with social work services, but in the training of the next generation of social workers, and in the policy-making of agencies. There will continue to be divided opinion about how relevant task-centred practice is to the wider citizen participation agenda (Croft and Beresford 1997; Payne 1997), but we believe that it can provide meaningful participation at the front line of services, with the potential to influence policies as well as practices. Not all people will be able, or wish, to participate at other levels of social work development, but every person has the right to expect full participation as a user of services. This is true even when the contact is not voluntary and not based on a shared view of what is wrong and what is needed.

Another area which enjoys strong support is the development of more collaborative learning and practice between the different professions (Barr 2002). Numerous inquiries have pointed to failures in understanding and communication between different professionals as key factors in the breakdown of services to protect people, usually children. Training courses are increasingly bringing students from different professions together in shared learning. As we hope to have demonstrated, task-centred practice is a method which can be used in work with a wide variety of individuals and groups in many different circumstances. Any individual professional, or team of different professionals, working with people experiencing personal or social problems can use the method. So far in the UK, task-centred practice has not moved much beyond social workers and social carers, but there is tremendous potential for the method to provide a common language of professional practice for a wide range of human services staff in health, education, social care and beyond.

There is a strong drive to develop 'evidence-based practice'. It is rather difficult to contemplate what practice could or should be based on, other than evidence, but the social work profession is right to focus on the need to be more curious about what kinds of social work practice work better than others, and in what circumstances; in the best sense of the word, to discriminate more carefully. Of course, the notion of 'evidence' is a contentious one. Some apply exceptionally narrow criteria; just when the physical sciences are getter softer (with chaos and quantum theories becoming more prominent), some would like the social sciences to harden. However, it is possible to argue for a more rigorous scrutiny of what makes for 'good practice' without subjecting every proposition to a randomised control test. Social work needs a form of practice which is systematic enough for comparisons and generalisations to be made with some confidence, yet flexible and practical enough to respond to an extraordinary variety of individual circumstances and limited resources; a form of practice which helps us work *with* the uncertainty rather than a pretence that we can control the uncertainty entirely or a resignation to a capricious world in which we can have no meaningful influence.

Task-centred practice makes the necessary compromises, and the evidence we have suggests that it *does* make a difference and that it invites systematic development. Each task-centred encounter is its own single case study, with a well-rounded view of 'evidence' which encompasses the experience and meaning of the work to those involved as well as judgements on the outcome. Each task-centred encounter derives from our collective learning from the past and builds towards our collective learning for the future.

TWELVE YEARS ON . . .

A dozen years lie between the publication of our first book on task-centred practice and this current one. In that time in the UK, the organisational and professional landscape has changed almost beyond recognition and the pace of change continues to quicken. For example, it is no longer a question of whether an organisation will restructure, but how many times. Things that were (social services departments, for instance) are, increasingly, no longer. Directives, targets, star ratings and the like are both symptom and cause of a strange kind of hyperactivity which is the current response to the shortfall between expectation and reality.

However, for the people who use social work services the scene is perhaps not so different now as it was in 1992. People still experience personal, interpersonal and social problems. There is still poverty and discrimination and large sections of our society are still marginalised and excluded.

There are other factors, too, which are not so changed:

- the need for a professional practice which is based on listening to people's concerns, harnessing their strengths and mobilising their resources
- the need for people who use social work services to contribute actively to developing and redeveloping them
- the need for practitioners who can recognise and articulate good practice, with the confidence to challenge poor practices and the ability to develop their own and others
- the need for a reasonably stable organisational and legislative context to support good practices.

If professional practice were to be developed and redeveloped in the ways we have been exploring in this book, what could the situation look like in 2016?

One of the few certainties is that people will continue to need the services which social workers can and should be providing. If task-centred practice were widely practised we would hope that, in addition to an increase in 'small successes' at the expense of 'large failures', we would also see the active accumulation of practice wisdom, systematically garnered, readily accessed and highly relevant. After all, it is the relevance of evidence which is likely to determine 'the ability and willingness of people to use it' (Fook *et al.* 2000: 192).

Access to local task planners, such as those developed by Reid (2000) based on the increasing and shared experience of task-centred encounters, would be hugely useful. Local compilations could network with regional and national 'Indexes', preserving confidentiality of course, all of which would link with other stores such as the electronic library for social care (eLSC). In this environment it would be the practice community to which policy makers would turn for advice and direction, and practitioners would become confident and expert at articulating good practice, over and above a set of general 'apple pie' principles. The organisations which employ social workers would benefit from this professional confidence and from the knowledge store which its workers and those who used its services were contributing.

In 2016, the uncertainty of practice, of course, remains undiminished. The search for a certain, risk-free practice is, at last, recognised as an illusion, and (ironically) a dangerous one which generates a proliferation of procedures and heavy-handed documentation, all of which take social workers away from their direct work with people. It is in this direct practice where uncertainty can best be worked with. The need to articulate a professional practice which meets these challenges, task-centred or not, is urgent.

APPENDIX

EXAMPLE ANSWERS TO SELECTED ACTIVITIES IN THE BOOK

ACTIVITY 1.2: Supervisor

Underpinning knowledge

How are you building your learning on the different strands that underpin task-centred practice? What systems do you use to search, appraise and store the following:

- legal knowledge
- research knowledge
- service user and carer views and experiences
- practice-based knowledge.

Do these areas all represent the same challenges to you regarding search, appraise and store?

Suggested answer

We all have systems for searching for knowledge, varying from a quick look at the bookshelf next to us to a systematic search via an electronic search engine. We appraise this material, possibly implicitly ('This looks reliable, it's from a well-known institution, and the author's previous work has been sound'), or maybe against criteria ('This is in a peer-reviewed journal'). We also all have systems for storing that knowledge, again varying enormously, from the pile on the floor to the colour-coded library boxes for different areas. Usually, and certainly in my case, these systems build up over time with not a great deal of conscious reflection about them. However, they are the key to success (although with an important caveat I will mention later) to coping with the mountain of knowledge there is out there: they will enable you to find material fast, to sort 'wheat from chaff', and to avoid storage taking up floor as well as wall space. Just reviewing them (i.e. searching, appraising, storing) for each of the areas above is well worthwhile, devoting time to this is genuinely time saved in the longer run, and crucial to a serious attempt to build up knowledge.

The only caveat about the importance of systems is that people can be just as, or more, important. The knowledgeable lawyer can save a vast amount of work finding legal knowledge, the knowledgeable research officer can do the same for research, and so on. An excellent librarian knows that however good the library catalogue or its search engines, a knowledgeable expert is nearly always the best at finding key information in their area. For each of the areas of knowledge above we try to have a number of people we know we can call on, and we deliberately try and build up and maintain this group.

A good help with searching and appraising is the research-mindedness website for social work (www.resmind.swap.ac.uk). It provides an excellent source of simple but sound training, advice and tools for doing search and appraisal work (including a useful self-assessment of your current skills).

A good help with storing information, including ideas about visual aids to do this and simple note ideas, can be found in Orna and Stevens' (1995) *Managing Information for Research*.

ACTIVITY 2.5: Practitioner

Keeping a log of problems and the tasks developed for them

When you start to develop your task-centred work, keep a log of the problems and the tasks that were developed for them. Over time you will be developing a personal task planner to remind you of the range of tasks that may be relevant, and as your work progresses and you can see which are more successful, you will be able to share some of the best ideas with other task-centred practitioners.

Suggested answer

Keeping a record of practice is not common. But a good gardener notes what grows in what site, a good photographer notes what scenes work best with which focal lengths, and so on. It is usual for people who are bothered about their expertise to try to find a structured way to record its development, to codify in some way their knowledge and skill development, and to record it for future use. It is not that common in social work. The lack of a language does not help, and all of the sections of this book that discuss practice development give a variety of other reasons that this is the case. Recording practice is therefore more difficult than it should be, there are not enough models, and there is not enough encouragement. However, the need to log work in 'continuing professional development' in order to maintain status as a registered social worker may help with changing the culture, as might the other issues raised in this book. The first stage, for me, in making sure I would do this log is to remind myself of its value, to make sure I reinforced my motivation to do this work. Task-centred work provides the language to do to the work. I would use a structure much like the one found in Reid's (2000) *Task Planner*. The first organising principle of the log is probably a problem classification, such as 'Alcoholism' through to 'Withdrawn child'. I would sort these categories out as I went, so that I could amalgamate or split them as needed. There is no universal problem framework to be applied at present. Then for each one I would make a quick note of the problem, and of any literature or other knowledge that I found particularly helpful. This would then be followed by the task I or others had developed and done (if successful, although a quick note of the unsuccessful ones may sometimes also be helpful).

Doing this systematically would be the best, but in the real world this will not happen often. Much like advice to dieters, that if you go for the chocolate cake once you should regard this as an aberration and not a reason to abandon your diet, the advice here is to accept that some weeks the log will be actively added to, and for other weeks nothing will occur. That's fine, reflecting on practice and building up practice knowledge may need to take second place to doing the practice, what should not happen is to lose it altogether.

ACTIVITY 3.2: MANAGER

Workload review: patterns of work

Do you have a clear idea of the workload levels for your staff? Is it possible for staff to undertake the 'short and fat' task-centred model of practice or do workload levels assume a 'long and thin' model? If more 'short and fat' work is to be done, will there be some recovery gaps between this more intensive work for staff to engage in learning or other activities?

Suggested answer

Workload levels are a constant issue, and judging them as a manager is constantly difficult. It is initially surprising how many people seem to have high workloads, and how few complain of underwork, but managers soon adjust to this version of reality! There are many models and practices for managing workload, the advice here is to make sure that practice sits at the heart of whatever practice is done. I would ask my staff about this, do the existing ways of handling workload really reflect the stresses of different parts of the work (for example, a point I will return to, beginnings are often harder than middle sections of work)? I would also ask them if the pattern of workload review or workload allocation can accommodate the 'short and fat' task-centred model. I would also do this via the team, to see how all views compared and to try to draw on all good ideas about how to help to promote workload models that can genuinely support practice, while being fair and reasonable to all.

The issue of 'recovery gaps' is important. As managers we often forget the different stresses of different parts of the work. Beginnings are usually harder, as people struggle to make sense of situations, and of course a more 'short and fat' model of practice has more beginnings. Allowance should be made for this. Also task-centred work is hard intellectual work, not just in terms of learning and developing (although including this in workload models is important) but also in terms of what is done in the sessions and in between. Working out 'SMART' goals is hard work, whereas agreeing 'fuzzy' ones is easier. Recognising this, and of course the payback there is to service users and carers of helping staff to cope with this extra work, is part of good management of task-centred practice.

ACTIVITY 4.3: TRAINER

Giving feedback from small groups to the large group

Feedback is an important aspect of most training programmes. However, there is the risk that it is repetitive and time-consuming, especially when a number of small groups have been working on the same task and are all asked to report back to each other.

- How would you organise feedback from the trios who have been rehearsing problem exploration in task-centred practice?
- What would you ask them to focus on?
- How would you avoid repetitiveness?

Suggested answer

I would consider how to organise the feedback so that it was interesting to the full group. Often, the feedback can become tedious because basically each group is pretty much saying the same thing. If there were five trios, I might ask each one to focus on different aspects of the problem exploration stage (e.g. the scan, additional problems, etc.).

The flipcharts could be used to break up the potential monotony of a stream of verbal feedbacks. Indeed, it would be useful to give each trio five minutes to organise their feedback – often we expect people just to think on their feet and you get a digest of what they've done and said rather than a reflection of their *learning* from the task. So, I would ask the trios to focus on the learning they have experienced rather than reporting on the content of the case.

To have some physical activity (they've probably been sitting down for a while), I might ask everyone to stand up and 'art gallery', that is physically move from one trio's flipchart to another.

ACTIVITY 5.5: LEARNER

Is it making a difference? Possible indicators

- How would you know whether your learning about task-centred practice is making a difference for the people you are working with? Make a note of some specific indicators that you and they could use to demonstrate the impact of this learning.
- How would you know whether your learning about task-centred practice is making a difference to your professional practice? Again, give some specific indicators which you and others could use.

Suggested answer

First, in terms of my learning making a difference with the people I am working with, I could use the task-centred record sheets to track this, but since these are solely concerned with the user or carer's progress, I would need to keep a reflective diary alongside them. Specific indicators could include:

- I used a particular technique (such as making 'headlines' on flipchart paper during the problem exploration phase) and the service user's feedback was positive.
- I negotiated a *written* agreement (which would be new to me), that it felt different, maybe even risky, but the service user evaluates it as an important part of the work.

Whatever the indicator, I guess I need to register the fact that it is 'new' in terms of new learning, but would want the impact on the service user or carer to be positive.

Second, in terms of my learning making a difference to my professional practice, I would look out for particular transfers of learning into my 'regular' practice. Examples of some specific indicators could include:

- I used more recording *in* sessions with people rather than writing about it afterwards.
- I found myself more able to reframe situations positively and to broaden my ability to recognise people's strengths.
- I am conscientious about conducting a thorough evaluation of work with service users rather than the usual 'How was it?'.
- I'm taking the messages from these evaluations into my practice, and feeding them into agency policies, too.

ACTIVITY 6.5: PRACTITIONER

Being specific

- We know that being specific increases the chances of success in resolving a problem. Choose one of the two examples of a selected problem (Boxes 6.3 and 6.4) and rewrite it so that it is more specific. Use your imagination to create additional information as appropriate.

Suggested answer

An improved example of Box 6.3.

EXAMPLE OF EXLORING PROBLEMS

Date of this session: 18 October
Persons involved: John (service user), Gwen (worker)
Problem chosen to work on (the selected problem):
'I used to have a right active, outgoing life; I can't get used to this now.'
Details of this problem:

What?

I find it very difficult to mix with other people and to experience new activities. This makes me very frustrated because I remember a life before my illness, when I was very active and outgoing.

Who?

It only affects me, though it's meant I've not seen my son for over four years, too. I guess that must affect him, too.

When?

This problem affects me every day. I have been living with it since I lost my driving school business and my family. Gradually over time I've become more and more isolated.

Where?

I now only feel comfortable going to the betting shop and the local market and I don't feel able to go anywhere else.

Why?

It is a problem because it restricts me. Also, there are things which I want to do which I can't do at present because of this problem. If I don't get social stimulation, my mind isn't active; doing maths puzzles and studying the form at the bookies helps subdue the problem by keeping my mind alert. If my mind isn't active, my problems get worse.

How?

It makes me feel bad about myself and I get into a spiral of no self-confidence.

Other problems included in the problem scan, but not being worked on at present:

Gwen feels that John's problem is related to his illness, though she acknowledges that he does not agree with her. Gwen feels that it can be a problem that John does not seek help from the psychiatrist or take the medication which he is prescribed. Again, she understands and agrees that this is also related to the problem of not having enough money (for prescriptions) and John's lack of confidence to go out to the chemist.

ACTIVITY 7.5: SERVICE USER AND CARER

Involving others in the work

The task-centred method encourages the involvement of other people who are directly involved in the problem or who are significant if the goal is going to be achieved.

- In what circumstances do you think other people should be involved in the review of your progress towards the goal? What can they contribute?
- In what circumstances might you not want this kind of involvement?

Suggested answer

If other people have been involved in helping me to achieve my goal, I can see that it would be good to have their viewpoint. They would be in a good position to comment because they would know what the goal was all about. This might be family members, or it could be other people that I'm involved with, such as the health visitor. Sometimes it gives you extra confidence when other people think you have done well, too. It would depend very much on what my goal was, and what I felt about these other people as to whether I felt they could contribute. I think it is a good idea if one of the last tasks is to find out from other people what they think about your achievements.

I would not want this kind of involvement if I did not trust that the person would be fair or honest. I would have to feel confident that they knew what to judge the goal against. Also, if my goal was a very personal and private one, I would expect the worker to respect this and not involve other people without my agreement.

ACTIVITY 8.1: MANAGER

What would an agency that has developed itself as a learning organisation look like?

Consider the organisation that you manage, and reflect on the following questions:

- Are there systems for reviewing the effectiveness of policy change and associated training?
- Does the policy and budget for training allow for a flexible development of learning, involving, for example, service users in change work?
- Are staff at all levels encouraged to play a role in development and change?
- Do teams allocate time for development, and do workload systems, as well as job descriptions, give recognition to development work?

Suggested answer

In a recent piece of work that one of the authors carried out for the Social Care Institute for Excellence, examples were sought of structures and processes which develop learning in an agency. Here are three examples. First, for one local authority, each year, a plan for development and training is devised from workforce and strategic analysis. This plan summarises the development needs of each service area and includes targets and budgets for achieving qualifications, for developing skills to meet new job requirements, for implementing changes, and for maintaining professional recognition.

Second, a group of learning disability service users have been trained as trainers and are paid a fee to lead consultation exercises, facilitate service development sessions and contribute to training programmes.

Third, in each service area a cross-section of staff form Training and Development Groups which meet regularly to plan, review and evaluate training and development activities. This has led, for example, to an audit of the training take-up by approved social workers, which identified and resolved many problems associated with training delivery and access.

ACTIVITY 8.4: SERVICE USER AND CARER

What would you expect from a task-centred worker?

Service users and carers might want to ask, as part of their analysis of the working partnership with social workers, what the skills, knowledge and experience are of the workers they are seeing. As a service user or carer, what answers would you expect from a task-centred worker?

Suggested answer

In the 1980s, in a piece of research on partnership-based practice, one of the authors had the following story relayed to him by a social worker who had, unusually for the decade in which the work took place, invited a father to a child protection conference that was about his child. The conference had begun with everyone introducing themselves and their jobs. After that the father had said:

> I'd like to ask one extra question of you all, please. I'm here because I am the father of the child you want to talk about, and I am here because I've known my child over all of his three years. Please would you each tell me what right you think you have to be here talking about my child, and how well you know that child?

There was a collective intake of breath.

It takes courage to do this, and of course the replies (and the issues they reflect) are really very complex; however, the point that all parties to social work actions should be able to say why they are there, and what knowledge they are bringing, is a vital one. I would expect a task-centred worker to be able to describe the mandate for being there, to be able to talk about skills in developing partnership (respect for others, communication skills, and so on), to be able to talk of knowledge about what helps people solve social problems (SMART goals, task development, and so on) and I would expect them to be honest about their experience ('I'm really new, but while that is a downside I do bring enthusiasm, and the latest training'). I want good answers to the questions about what the partnership is and what skills, knowledge and experience social workers bring to this partnership.

REFERENCES

Ahmad, B. (1990) *Black Perspectives in Social Work* Birmingham: Venture Press

Alibhai-Brown, Y. (2001) *Who Do We Think We Are? Imagining the New Britain* London: Penguin

Atherton, C. (1982) The task force *Social Work Today* 14, 2: 8–10

Atkins, J. (2002) The emotional dimension of learning *Learning in Health and Social Care* 1, 1: 61–62

Barnes, M. and Bowl, R. (2001) *Taking Over the Asylum* Basingstoke: Palgrave

Barr, H. (2002) *Interprofessional Education: Today, Yesterday and Tomorrow* London: Learning and Teaching Support Network for Health Sciences and Practice

Bricker-Jenkins, M. (1990) Another approach to practice and training: clients must be considered the primary experts *Public Welfare* 48, 2: 11–16

Brodie, I. (1993) Teaching from practice in social work education: a study of the content of supervision sessions *Issues in Social Work Education* 13, 2: 71–91

Brown, L. B. (1977) Treating problems of psychiatric outpatients. In *Task-Centred Practice* W. J. Reid and L. Epstein (eds). New York: Columbia University Press

Butler, J., Bow, I. and Gibbons, J. (1978) Task-centred casework with marital problems *British Journal of Social Work* 8: 393–409

Caspi, J. and Reid, W. J. (2002) *Educational Supervision in Social Work: A Task-centered Model for Field Instruction and Staff Development* New York: Columbia University Press

Clare, M. (1988) Supervision, role strain and social services departments *British Journal of Social Work* 18: 489–507

Clarke, J., Gerwitz, S. and McLauglin, E. (eds) (2000) *New Managerialism, New Welfare* London: Sage Publications

Cree, V. and Macaulay, C. (eds) (2000) *Transfer of Learning in Professional and Vocational Education* London: Routledge

Croft, S. and Beresford, P. (1997) Service users' perspectives. In M. Davies (ed) *The Blackwell Companion to Social Work* Oxford: Blackwell

Davies, C. (1998) The cloak of professionalism. In M. Allot and M. Robb (eds) *Understanding Health and Social Care: An Introductory Reader* London: Sage Publications

Davies, M. (ed) (2000) *The Blackwell Encyclopaedia of Social Work* Oxford: Blackwell

de Bono, E. (2000) *Six Hat Thinking* London: Penguin

Dean, R. G. (1998) A narrative approach to groups *Clinical Social Work Journal* 26, 1: 23–37

Department of Health (2000) *Framework for the Assessment of Children in Need and their Families* London: The Stationery Office

Department of Health (2002) *National Service Framework for Older People: Single Assessment Process* London: The Stationery Office

Department of Health (2004) Social work careers (www.socialworkcareers.co.uk)

Dierking, B., Brown, M. and Fortune, A. E. (1980) Task-centred treatment in a residential facility for the elderly: a clinical trial *Journal of Gerontological Social Work* 2(spring): 225–240

Doel, M. and Marsh, P. (1992) *Task-centred Social Work* Aldershot: Ashgate

Doel, M. and Marsh, P. (1995) Task-Centred Portfolio. A template portfolio used by participants in the Task-Centred Practice accredited training programme, Wakefield.

Doel, M., Sawdon, C. and Morrison, D. (2002) *Learning, Practice and Assessment: Signposting the Portfolio* London: Jessica Kingsley

Dominelli, L. (1996) Deprofessionalising social work: anti-oppressive practice, competencies and post-modernism *British Journal of Social Work* 26: 153–175

Drath, W. H. and Palus, C. J. (1994) *Making Common Sense: Leadership as Meaning-making in a Community of Practice* Greensboro, NC: Center for Creative Leadership

Egan, G. (1986) *The Skilled Helper* Pacific Grove, CA: Brooks/Cole

Encarta (1999) *World English Dictionary* London: Bloomsbury

Eraut, M. (2004) The emotional content of learning: editorial *Learning in Health and Social Care* 3, 1: 1–4

Fisher, M. and Marsh, P. (2003) Social work research and the 2001 Research Assessment Exercise: an initial overview *Social Work Education* 22, 1: 71–80

Fook, J., Ryan, M. and Hawkins, L. (2000) *Professional Expertise: Practice, Theory and Education for Working in Uncertainty* London: Whiting and Birch

Fortune, A. E. (ed) (1985) *Task-Centred Practice with Families and Groups* New York: Springer

Gallwey, W. T. (1986) *The Inner Game of Tennis* London: Pan

Garvin, C. (1985) Practice with task-centred groups. In A. E. Fortune (ed) *Task-Centred Practice with Families and Groups* New York: Springer

General Social Care Council (2002) *Code of Practice for Social Care Workers and for Employers of Social Care Workers* London: General Social Care Council

Gibbons, J. S., Bow, I., Butler, J. and Powell, J. (1979) Clients' reactions to task-centred casework: a follow-up study *British Journal of Social Work* 9: 203–215

Gibbons, J., Bow, I. and Butler, J. (1984) Task-centred work after parasuicide. In E. M. Goldberg, J. Gibbons and I. Sinclair (eds) *Problems, Tasks and Outcomes: The Evaluation of Task-Centred Casework* London: Allen and Unwin

Gibbons, J. S., Butler, J., Urwin, P. and Gibbons, J. L. (1978) Evaluation of a social work service for self-poisoning patients *British Journal of Psychiatry* 133: 111–118

Gingerich, W. J. and Eisengart, S. (2000) Solution-focused brief therapy: a review of the outcome research *Family Process* 39, 4: 477–498

Goldberg, E.M., Gibbons, J. and Sinclair, I. (eds) (1984a) *Problems, Tasks and Outcomes: The Evaluation of Task-centred Casework in Three Settings* NISW Library 47, London: Allen and Unwin

Goldberg, E. M. and Stanley, S. J. with Kenrick, A. (1984b) Task-centred casework in a probation setting. In E. M. Goldberg, J. Gibbons and I. Sinclair (eds) *Problems, Tasks and Outcomes: The Evaluation of Task-Centred Casework in Three Settings* London: Allen and Unwin

Greene, J. and Grant, A. M. (2003) *Solution-Focused Coaching* London: Pearson Education

Howard, G. S. (1991) Culture tales: a narrative approach to thinking, cross-cultural psychology, and psychotherapy *American Psychologist* 46, 3: 187–197

Iles, V. and Sutherland, K. (2001) *Organisational Change: A Review for Health Care Managers, Professionals and Researchers* London: National Co-ordinating Centre for NHS Service Delivery and Organisation R & D

Isaacs, D. and Fitzgerald, D. (1999) Seven alternatives to evidence-based medicine *British Medical Journal* 319: 1618

Kearney, T. (1998) The contribution of observation to management in the personal social services. In P. Le Riche and K. Tanner (eds) *Observation and its Application to Social Work* London: Jessica Kingsley

Kirk, S. A. and Reid, W. J. (2002) *Science and Social Work: A Critical Appraisal* New York: Columbia University Press

Larsen, J. and Mitchell, C. T. (1980) Task-centred strength-oriented group work with delinquents *Social Casework* 61(March): 154–163

Le Riche, P. and Tanner, K. (eds) (1998) *Observation and its Application to Social Work – Rather Like Breathing* London: Jessica Kingsley

Lewis, J. (2001) What works in community care? *Managing Community Care* 9, 1: 3–6

Lewis, J. (2002) The contribution of research findings to practice change *MCC Building Knowledge for Integrated Care* 10, 1: 9–12

Maalouf, A. (2000) On Identity London: Harvill Press

McCartt Hess, P. and Mullen, E. J. (1995) *Practitioner–Researcher Partnerships* Washington, DC: NASW Press

McCaughan, N. and Vickery, A. (1982) Staging the play *Social Work Today* 14, 2: 11–13

Macy-Lewis, J. A. (1985) Single parent groups. In A. E. Fortune (ed) *Task-Centred Practice with Families and Groups* New York: Springer

Marsh, P. (1990) Changing practice in child care – the Children Act 1989 *Adoption and Fostering* 14, 4: 27–30

Marsh, P. and Fisher, M. (1992) *Good Intentions: Developing Partnership in Social Services* York: Joseph Rowntree Foundation

Marsh, P. and Triseliotis, J. (1996) *Ready to Practise? Social Workers and Probation Officers: Their Training and First Year in Work* Aldershot: Avebury

Naleppa, M. J. and Reid, W. J. (1998) Task-centred case management for the elderly: developing a practice model *Research on Social Work Practice* 8, 1: 63–85

Newton, C. and Marsh, P. (1993) *Training in Partnership: Translating Intentions into Practice in Social Services* York: Joseph Rowntree Foundation

O'Hagan, K. (2001) *Cultural Competence in the Caring Professions* London: Jessica Kingsley

Orna, E. and Stevens, G. (1995) *Managing Information for Research* Buckingham: Open University Press

Parihar, B. (1984) *Task-Centred Management in Human Services* Springfield, IL: Charles C. Thomas

Parsloe, E. and Wray, M. (2000) *Coaching and Mentoring* London: Kogan Page

Payne, C. and Scott, T. (1982) *Developing Supervision of Teams in Field and Residential Social Work* London: National Institute for Social Work

Payne, M. (1997) Task-centred practice within the politics of social work theory *Issues in Social Work Education* 17, 2: 48–65

Pedler, M. and Aspinwall, K. (1998) *A Concise Guide to the Learning Organization* London: Lemos & Crane

Pichot, T. and Dolan, Y. M. (2003) *Solution-Focused Brief Therapy* Binghamton, NY: Haworth Clinical Practice Press

Pithouse, A. (1998) *Social Work: The Social Organisation of an Invisible Trade* Aldershot: Avebury

Rathbone-McCuan, E. (1985) Intergenerational family practice with older families. In A. E. Fortune (ed) *Task-Centred Practice with Families and Groups* New York: Springer

Reid, W. J. (1963) *An Experimental Study of Methods Used in Casework Treatment* New York: Columbia University School of Social Work

Reid, W. J. (1975) A test of a task-centred approach *Social Work* 20 (January): 3–9

Reid, W. J. (1992) *Task Strategies: An Empirical Approach to Social Work* New York: Columbia University Press

Reid, W. J. (1997) Research on task-centred practice *Research in Social Work* 21, 3: 132–137

Reid, W. J. (2000) *The Task Planner: An Intervention Resource for Human Service Planners* New York: Columbia University Press

Reid, W. J. and Epstein, L. (1972) *Task-Centred Casework* New York: Columbia University Press

Reid, W. J. and Shyne, A. W. (1969) *Brief and Extended Casework* New York: Columbia University Press

Richards, M. and Payne, C. with Shepperd, A. (1990) *Staff Supervision in Child Protection Work* London: National Institute for Social Work

Rogers, E. M. (1995) *Diffusion of Innovations* New York: The Free Press

Rooney, R. H. (1981) A task-centred reunification model for foster care. In A. N. Maluccio and P. A. Sinanoglu (eds) *The Challenge of Partnership: Working with Parents of Children in Foster Care* New York: Child Welfare League of America

Rooney, R. H. (1988) Measuring task-centred training effects on practice: results of an audiotape study in a public agency *Journal of Continuing Social Work Education* 4, 4: 2–7

Rooney, R. H. (1992) *Strategies for Work with Involuntary Clients* New York: Columbia University Press

Rushton, A. and Martyn, H. (1990) Two post-qualifying courses in social work: the views of the course members and their employers *British Journal of Social Work* 20: 445–468

Rzepnicki, T. L. (1982) *Task-Centred Intervention: An Adaptation and Test of Effectiveness in Foster Care Services* Chicago, IL: University of Chicago

Schön, D. (1987) *Educating the Reflective Practitioner* San Francisco, CA: Josey-Bass

Shaw, I. and Lishman, J. (eds) (1999) *Evaluation and Social Work Practice*. London: Sage Publications

Shemmings, D. (1991) *Client Access to Records: Participation in Social Work* Aldershot: Avebury

Smale, G. D. (1983) Can we afford not to develop social work practice? *British Journal of Social Work* 13: 251–264

Smale, G. D. (1996) *Mapping Change and Innovation* London: HMSO

Smale, G. D. (1998) *Managing Change through Innovation* London: The Stationery Office

Stepney, P. and Ford, D. (2000) *Social Work Models, Methods and Theories: A Framework for Practice* Lyme Regis, UK: Russell House

Stocking, B. (1985) *Initiative and Inertia: Case Studies in the NHS* London: Nuffield Provincial Hospitals Trust

Streatfield, D. and Wilson, T. (1980) *The Vital Link: Information in Social Services Departments* Sheffield: Joint Unit for Social Services Research, University of Sheffield

Tolson, E. R. and Reid, W. J. (eds) (1981) *Models of Family Treatment* New York: Columbia University Press

Tolson, E., Reid, W. J. and Garvin, C. D. (1994) *Generalist Practice: A Task-Centered Approach* New York: Columbia University Press

Trevithick, P. (2000) *Social Work Skills* Buckingham: Open University Press

Trinder, L. (2000) Evidence-based practice in social work and probation. In L. Trinder and S. Reynolds (eds) *Evidence-based Practice: A Critical Appraisal* Oxford: Blackwell Science

Turner, M. and Evans, C. (2004) Users influencing the management of practice. In D. Statham (ed) *Managing Front Line Practice in Social Care* London: Jessica Kingsley

Verbeek, G. (1997) Combining client interests with professionalism in the organisation. In A. Evers, R. Haverinen, K. Leichsenring and G. Wistow (eds) *Developing Quality in Personal Social Services: Concepts, Cases and Comments* Aldershot: Ashgate

Wedenoja, M., Nurius, P. and Tripodi, T. (1988) Enhancing mindfulness in practice prescriptive thinking *Social Casework* 69, 7: 427–433

Weingarten, K. (1998) The small and the ordinary: the daily practice of a postmodern narrative therapy *Family Process* 37: 3–15

Wenger, E. (1998) *Communities of Practice* Cambridge: Cambridge University Press

Wenger, E., McDermott, R. and Snyder, W. M. (2002) *Cultivating Communities of Practice* Cambridge, MA: Harvard Business School Press

Wilson, K. (2002) *The Single Assessment Process and Easycare* Sheffield: University of Sheffield

Yelloly, M. and Henkel, M. (1995) *Learning and Teaching in Social Work: Towards Reflective Practice* London: Jessica Kingsley

WEBSITES

Department of Health – www.socialworkcareers.co.uk
Easycare – www.sheffield.ac.uk/sisa/easycare
Electronic Library for Social Care (eLSC) – www.elsc.org.uk Social Care Institute for Excellence, London.
Research-mindedness for Social Work – www.resmind.swap.ac.uk

INDEX